HEIDEGGER, MEDICINE
& 'SCIENTIFIC METHOD'

HEIDEGGER, MEDICINE & 'SCIENTIFIC METHOD'

The Unheeded Message of the Zollikon Seminars

Peter Wilberg

New Gnosis Publications

2nd edition 2018 published by **New Yoga Publications**
First published by **New Gnosis Publications**
www.newgnosis.co.uk

ISBN 1-904519-03-2

CONTENTS

Preface

This book draws on Heidegger's reflections on science as 'method' to introduce a new phenomenological concept of 'scientific method'. Phenomenology is not presented simply as an alternative method of qualitative scientific research of particular or exclusive relevance to the human sciences, but as the basis of any truly *fundamental science* – and of a fundamentally new understanding of *medicine* in particular. The book is in five parts:

Part 1 deals with the underlying aims and assumptions of the 'modern scientific method', with particular emphasis on their application in modern medicine. Its primary sources are the central issues raised by Heidegger with physicians and psychiatrists in the course of the *Zollikon Seminars*.

It also addresses the fundamental nature of modern science as a sense-making or 'semiotic' activity, one that seeks ordered patterns of significance in phenomena. The semiotics of modern science is contrasted with an authentic phenomenological semiotics – one that does not *reduce* the meaning of phenomena to their place within already established patterns of significance.

Part 2 seeks to show how a *field-dynamic* concept of 'phenomenology' can lay the foundations of a new *field-phenomenological medicine* - one that transcends the metaphysical and methodological assumption of current medical science and practice. It begins with a summary of the basic principles of field-phenomenological science and goes on to explore different phenomenological, ontological, relational and cultural dimensions of medical theory and practice.

Part 3 explores the *ethical-historical dimensions* of biological and genetic medicine, in particular the links between eugenics and human genomics and the key role played by German physicians and psychiatrists in providing a 'medical-model' justification for scapegoating all people of Jewish ancestry. In doing so it acknowledges Heidegger's role in challenging what he called Hitler's "biological materialism" as well as biological and genetic medicine in general.

Part 4 sets out the practical essence of field-phenomenological medicine as *meta-medicine* or 'medicine beyond medicine' – a new *existential* approach to health and healing grounded in three fundamental ontological distinctions: between the human *body* and the human *being*, between the physical body (*Körper*) and the felt or lived body (*Leib*), and between the clinical manifestations of *disease pathology* on the one hand and, on the other hand, the felt *dis-ease* or *pathos* which it embodies.

Part 5 outlines in a new way the basic principles of the *phenomenological method*, doing so in a manner that highlights its relevance for both the human and natural sciences. It is the author's belief that phenomenological method, understood as the essence of scientific method *per se*, fulfils not only the original scientific project of Husserlian phenomenology but also Marx's humanistic vision of a unified or "integral" science - one that is both a "natural science of man" and a "human science of nature".

Heidegger and Scientific Method

Let us first of all deconstruct what might be termed the myth of 'scientific method' as this is currently understood: a set of rational procedures guaranteed to eliminate mere dogma from "true" scientific knowledge, distinguish empirical fact from mere belief or hypothesis. So what exactly is the modern scientific "method" - that veritable barricade of investigative procedures designed to defend institutionalized science from empty supposition or pseudo-science? Modern scientific method understands itself as a five-stage process involving:

1. Observation and description of a phenomenon.
2. Formulation of a hypothesis that explains the phenomenon.
3. Use of the hypothesis to predict other phenomena.
4. Controlled experiments designed to test these predictions.
5. Validation of their results by independent researchers.

The first and most important questions raised by this self-definition are those it notably fails to address. The questions are:

1. What *counts* as a phenomenon in the first place?
2. What *account* is given of the phenomenon itself?
3. In what ways can the phenomenon be *accounted* for?

These questions are of fundamental methodological significance, for as Heidegger points out: "All explanation reaches only so far as the explication of that which is to be explained."

Heidegger himself gives several examples of phenomena to which the questions apply, amongst them "grief and tears". Before we can formulate and confirm a 'scientific' hypothesis to explain the phenomenon of 'tears' for example, we must first ask ourselves what the phenomenon itself essentially is. Within the modern scientific method however, what *counts* as a phenomenon is above all that which is countable - measurable. To which Heidegger counters: "In reality you can never measure tears; rather when you measure, it is at best a fluid and its drops that you measure, but not tears."

Are tears a somatic phenomenon, a psychical phenomenon or a 'psychosomatic' phenomenon - the somatic effect of a psychical phenomenon such as 'grief'? If so, does that mean that the somatic fluid drops produced by an irritated and watering eye are just as much tears as those produced by a person weeping in grief, i.e. essentially the same phenomenon except with a different 'cause'? The fact that 'scientifically' speaking, we refer to 'tear ducts' as physiological givens, implies as much. The physiological designation sets aside the fundamental methodological question of what constitutes the phenomenon of tears as such - in distinction from other phenomena such as over-watering eyes. Before any possible hypotheses can be vouched or experiments ventured, therefore, the modern scientific method has already given its own dogmatic answers to the three fundamental methodological questions:

1. What *counts* as a phenomenon is only that which we can observe outwardly - measurable fluid drops produced by the eyes.
2. Our *account* of what tears are as a phenomenon will make no distinction between weeping in grief and watering eyes.
3. We can *account* for tears only by suggesting mechanisms of either physiological or 'psychosomatic' *causation*.

What possible experiment however, could be devised that would provide 'reliable' quantitative evidence of a *causal* relation between a psychic state such as grief and its somatic expression in tears? We would first of all have to be in a position to 'measure' grief. Heidegger again: "How does one measure grief? One obviously can't measure it at all. Why not? Were one to apply a method of measurement to grief we would offend against the meaning of grief and would have already ruled out in advance the grief as grief. The very attempt to measure would offend against the phenomenon as phenomenon."

Heidegger goes on to emphasise that the fact that we speak of someone grieving less or more intensely, does not mean we are speaking of a measurable quantity of grief, but rather of its quality. We are referring to qualitative depth and intensity. As for the tears that can supposedly be accounted for as something 'caused' by grief, we are once again offending against the phenomenon as phenomenon. Tears as tears - as expressions of sadness or unhappiness, pain or grief are not a physical phenomenon that we first observe and then account for, scientifically or otherwise. We do not first see drops of water in a person's eyes, then conclude, from the circumstance, that they are grieving and therefore understand them to be weeping in grief. The immediately observed phenomenon is not fluid drops in a person's eyes but *a person weeping* - not an isolated physical perception but a perceptual whole or gestalt. It is only through *abstraction* from this gestalt - from the phenomenon as a phenomenon - that we arrive at an account of what 'tears' are that reduce them to something 'psychical' *or* 'somatic'. An account of the phenomenon that then demands explanatory accounting for in terms of some 'mechanism' of psychosomatic 'causation'.

Heidegger goes on to question how things stand with the phenomenon of pain, comparing for example the pain of grief with bodily pain of some sort.

"How do things stand regarding both these 'pains'? Are both somatic or both psychical, or is only the one somatic and the other psychical, or are both pains neither one nor the other?"

Any account we might give in such terms of pain as a phenomenon, or any typology of pain phenomena we might construct - distinguishing somatic and emotional pain, real and imaginary pain etc. would both immediately foreclose the question of what the phenomenon itself - *pain as such* - essentially is. But the question of what pain itself essentially is and how it can be accounted for is not the object of any possible experiment. It is first and foremost a question of what it means to us to 'be in pain' i.e. the different ways (mental, emotional and physical) in which we are aware of *being* in pain, and the different ways in which we interpret, emotionalise and embody pain as a state of *being*.

The modern scientific method rules out in advance as possible objects of scientific investigation all phenomena that cannot be reduced to observable and measurable sensory 'phenomena' such as 'tear' drops or electrical 'pain' signals.

In doing so it rules out any genuinely empirical approach to phenomena as such - any exploration of the way we actually experience those phenomena. But that is precisely the task of any genuinely empirical, genuinely phenomenological science.

Whilst science is itself a human activity which assumes the existence of aware human beings capable of creating hypotheses and testing them through experimental observations and measurements, the modern scientific method cannot so much as prove the existence of single human being - as opposed to a talking body-object. Nor can it provide evidence for a single state of being such as love or fear, grief or pain, joy or sadness, or for the scientist's own taken-for-granted awareness of the world - the condition for their observation and measurement of any phenomenon whatsoever. After all, from a physical-scientific viewpoint, instruments can be used to measure and observe things without us assuming any awareness on their part - so the same applies to the scientists using those instruments. From a modern scientific point of view, as Heidegger put it quite simply: "One cannot prove that one exists."

What we are left with then, is a 'method' which seeks 'scientific' explanations for phenomena but at the same time:

- forgets that awareness is the *condition* for our observation and measurement of any phenomena whatsoever
- either takes our awareness of phenomena for granted or seeks to *reduce* this awareness to one phenomenon amongst others
- is based on *unverifiable* postulations of physical energies and entities inaccessible to direct awareness

- is unable, in principle, to explain how awareness can arise within a fundamentally *unaware* universe of matter and energy
- *assumes* the scientist's own awareness of phenomena without 'proving' this awareness or questioning the view of phenomena it presents

One might ask how such a blatantly self-contradictory concept of scientific 'truth' and scientific 'method' managed to ever justify itself. It has done so by maintaining the myth that awareness or subjectivity is essentially private property. Because of this, subjective experience and subjective phenomena are seen as essentially unverifiable, whereas what science deals with is an 'outer' world of objective, publicly verifiable phenomena - one supposedly independent of subjectivity and of a private 'inner' world of subjective experience and phenomena.

Husserl was the first modern thinker to put into question this dualistic world outlook - pointing out that subjectivity or awareness is not a separate domain, a sealed and private inner world, but that which first makes it possible to experience an 'outer' world at all. What we experience 'out there' in the world consists just as much of phenomena we experience and interpret subjectively as anything we might experience in the inner world of our dreams.

Conversely, that which science regards as 'purely' subjective phenomena of the sort not amenable to direct 'empirical' investigation - dreams and desires, love and hate, pain and pleasure, grief and joy - are (at least for the great mass of mankind unschooled in the modern scientific method) not sealed off private experiences but shared and public realities. In this shared and public world what we see is not fluid drops exuded from tear ducts under certain conditions - we see people *crying* or *holding back tears*. We see the as yet invisible and immeasurable tears they hold back no less than the visible and potentially measurable tears they shed. In other words we see tears, the empirical phenomena as such and not some scientific abstraction from it.

What is known in academic circles as "phenomenology" - that intimidating, and for many almost unpronounceable, mouthful of a word, is not some marker or footnote in the history of philosophy. Nor is it merely one approach amongst others vaunted within academic disciplines called 'philosophy' or 'philosophy of science'. The term phenomenology designates the fundamental essence of science and scientific method as such - the essence of any genuinely fundamental science. The 'phenomenological method' is scientific method properly understood. By contrast, what passes as 'method' today in the physical sciences is, as Heidegger put it "through and through dogmatic; dealing with un-thought-through conceptions and preconceptions". Indeed, it stands on a par with fundamentalist religious dogmas. The latter are used as a standard for determining the credibility and religious acceptability of other beliefs, religious and scientific. The modern scientific method is also a set of beliefs used to determine the credibility and 'scientific' acceptability of other beliefs. The phenomenological method is not a body of beliefs. It is based on the suspension or 'bracketing' of all beliefs and preconceptions. Therefore its starting point is not and cannot be a preconceived division of phenomena into two domains of experience: 'objective' and 'subjective', 'outer' and 'inner', 'public' and 'private'. Nor does it begin by 'bracketing off' the entire realm of 'inner experience', treating it as something purely 'private' and therefore not capable of methodical scientific research.

The unquestioned assumptions that lie at the basis of Western science and find expression in the five-stage procedure previously outlined stand in contrast to the phenomenological approach adopted within Eastern spiritual traditions. Here disciplined meditational procedures were employed as methodically as modern experimental procedures - not simply in order to come up with models of observed relationships *between* experienced phenomena, but in order to alter the researcher's customary relationship to those phenomena and thereby deepen and enrich their direct experience of them. Neither the meditational knowledge-seeker nor the modern experimental researcher starts out with a Cartesian attitude of doubting everything. Instead their training requires them to accept 'on faith' an institutionalized body of knowledge. The latter, which already determines what 'counts' as significant phenomena, already provides an account of the essential nature of these phenomena, and of the underlying 'laws' they conform to.

The idea that *meditational* research deals with a realm of private psychic experience about which no communal scientific consensus can be established is given the lie by the sheer sophistication of the bodies of knowledge that have grown up around the spiritual traditions of the East - albeit a knowledge couched in terms radically different from the theoretical jargons of the modern sciences. These evolving bodies of 'spiritual' knowledge have also gone through their own major 'paradigm shifts' - and remain no less in need of continuous refinement and reinterpretation than do the models and terminologies of modern science.

The modern scientific method has replaced meditative enquiry and meditational research with mathematics. This is a paradox in itself, for despite the dominant role played by mathematics in physical scientific explanations of phenomena, the truth of mathematical *reasoning* is not itself anything for which evidence can be found in those phenomena. As McFarlane points out: "The Pythagorean theorem, for example, is and will always be true regardless of any sensory experiences." Experimental data may confirm or invalidate a particular mathematical model. But the internal coherence of the model and of mathematical reasoning in general is founded, like logical reasoning is founded, on 'subjective' intuition not objective fact. This is a type of intuition that is lent great precision by mathematical training in the formal methods of mathematic reasoning. Similarly, meditative intuition can be lent great precision by training in both methods of meditation and of meditative thinking as such.

Fundamental research, as phenomenological research, is not *mathematical* but is essentially *methodical* and *meditative* in nature. For Husserl the essence of the phenomenological method lay in 'bracketing' the whole idea of a world of pre-given phenomena whose inter-relationships can be studied independently of our own aware relationship to them - the modes of relatedness and modes of awareness in which they first come to presence as phenomena. For Heidegger what was decisive in the phenomenological method was the principle, already quoted, that all explanation of a phenomenon reaches only so far as our explication of the phenomena - our understanding of what it is we are seeking an explanation for. Phenomenological science does not begin by formulating explanatory hypotheses, for this is to assume, without further ado, that we already know what the phenomenon under investigation essentially is. Heidegger himself uses the now highly pertinent and topical example of the phenomenon of illness and its genetic explanation of its aetiology:

"The significance, indeed, the necessity of the genetic approach is clear to everyone. It seems self-evident. But it suffers from a deficit, which is all too easily and therefore all too often overlooked. To be in a position to explain an illness genetically, we need first of all to explain what the illness in itself is. It can be that a true understanding of the essence of an illness...prohibits all causal-genetic explanation....Those who wish to stick rigidly to genetic explanation, without first of all clarifying the essence of that which they wish to explain, can be compared to people who wish to reach a goal, without first of all bringing this goal in view."

There are more and more people today who do indeed question the medical-scientific assumption that illness is a purely biological phenomenon with an 'organic' or 'genetic' basis. Instead they see illness as something that does not merely have a specific cause in the human body but a specific meaning for the human being. They understand that the felt experience of illness and its felt meaning for the individual is no mere symptomatic or social by-product of physiological processes or 'disorders' but rather belongs to its very essence as a phenomenon. A phenomenological investigation of illness would explore the close relation between illness and identity, the felt body and our felt sense of self, our immune system and its defences and the mental defences we erect to preserve a singular stable sense of identity.

It may seem unfair to use medicine and psychology rather than physics to focus on the contrast between physical science and its methods on the one hand, and the phenomenological method on the other. But throughout his critical analysis of the modern scientific method, Heidegger emphasized the intimate relation between modern conceptions of method and modern conceptions of *bodyhood*. Tracing the modern scientific method back to its first formulation in the philosophy of Descartes, Heidegger sees its foundation in the Cartesian concept of a disembodied subject or 'ego', separate and independent of its objects, which makes the self-certainty of its own independent reality ("I think therefore I am") and its own mathematical reasoning into the measure of all things. That this disembodied ego happens to be mysteriously located in some physical body object only confirms its own separation from those other bodies that are the objects of physical-scientific investigation. Out of this concept comes a 'scientific' definition of truth which rules out in advance all that cannot be quantitatively measured and calculatively predicted with the highest degree of mathematical certainty or probability. The root meaning of the word phenomenon is *phainesthai* – to shine forth or come to light. The purpose of the modern scientific method is not, as in Greek to let phenomena show themselves or come to light in their essential nature, but rather to *secure* with maximum calculative certainty the reckonability, predictability and controllability of both nature and man.

Modern 'scientific method' is in this sense the credo of what today has been termed the 'control freak'. Calculation and control, however, are themselves a specific mode of relatedness to the world. But this mode of relatedness to the world, that governs the methical scientific procedures of the physicist, chemist or biologist is not itself anything physical, chemical or biological, nor is it the object of any possible experiment. It is a way of being in the world in which the researcher's mental attitude is all important but in which the scientist's felt bodily relation to space and time, things and people, has no place. For the human body itself is seen as a physical body-object no different in essence from any other.

The scientist takes the standpoint that their own "I" is here, whilst the object, whether thing or person, is 'over there' or 'out there', to be viewed at a distance through the lens of some body organ or instrument. Phenomenologically understood, things are quite different, however. Our "being-in-the-world" is not a composite of three discrete elements: an ego or "I", a body-object, and the world understood as a set of other body-objects. For our being 'here' is at the same time a being 'there' *with*, and as I will suggest *within* those other body objects.

"When I direct someone towards a windowsill with a gesture of my right hand, my bodily existence as a human being does not end at the tip of my index finger. While perceiving the windowsill....I extend myself bodily far beyond this fingertip to that windowsill. In fact, bodily I reach out even further than this to touch all the phenomena, present or merely visualized, represented ones."

What appears as the physical phenomenon of space is the space of our own bodily awareness of the world. The space of our body's sensory awareness of the world has a *non-local* or field character - it is not bounded by the spatial dimensions of our own bodies viewed as *localized* objects within that space. Fundamental science is *field-phenomenological* science, dispensing with the notion that subjectivity or awareness is something localized within objects in physical space (the human brain for example) and recognizing instead its own intrinsic spatiality, its non-local or field character.

The second major principle of the phenomenological method as Heidegger presents it, is awareness of our own mode of relatedness to things, our way of "being-in-the world". But there is no way of being in the world, not even that of the model modern scientist, that is not grounded in a particular relation to our own bodies, and to our own felt, bodily relation to the world. The question for Heidegger is only whether we fully *let ourselves into* this felt bodily relation to the world, whether we become aware of it or whether we reduce our own bodyhood to a mere object for a disembodied subject or "I", an object that is in 'space' in the manner of a physical object. Heidegger challenges the whole idea that our own bodies stand 'in' space in the same way that a glass of water stands on a table, that they are seated on chairs in the same way that a cushion might be, or that they move in essentially the same manner as billiard balls. It is not my body that rests on the chair upon which I sit. I rest on the seat in a bodily way. My seatedness, like my potential movements in space, and like my perception of other objects in space, are not states, actions or perceptions of an independent body-object. They are different ways in which I *body* my own being in the world. But as Heidegger points out:

"We know by now a great deal - almost more than we can encompass - about what we call the body, without having seriously thought about what bodying is. It is something more and different from merely 'carrying a body around with one'."

The modern scientific method is itself the *embodiment* of a particular way of being in the world, and of a particular mode of relatedness, not only to the world, but to our own bodies. It was in the course of the nineteenth century that this method firmly established itself. But as Nietzsche already recognized at the time: "It is not the victory of *science* that characterizes our 19th century, but the victory of scientific *method* over science." Quoting this statement of Nietzsche's, Heidegger adds, that for this method, what is primary is "not nature, as it addresses itself to mankind…but how mankind, with the intention of conquering nature should represent nature to itself." It is "the most monstrous assault of mankind on nature". The conclusion from these remarks is a simple one. Science is not something to be abandoned to superstition, substituted for with the symbols of archaic spiritual traditions, or sacrificed to the demands of corporate profit-making. Nor, however, is it something that can any more be left to those scientists, who, as disciples of the modern scientific method, remain in bondage to their own dogmas. In doing so they have reduced themselves to the status of corporate servants, paid to dish up an endless supply of new technologies with which not only nature but our own human nature - our bodies themselves - can be psychologically, chemically and genetically assaulted, all in the holy name of 'science'.

Nowhere is *this* subservient role of the modern scientific method better illustrated than in the use of so-called "Controlled Clinical Studies" to test new medical and psychiatric drugs or treatments. Even before they have begun, the 'scientific method' behind these studies has already reduced the individual patient to a case of some pre-defined generic disease, has reduced their felt dis-ease or discomfort to a checklist of pre-defined symptoms which can be ticked off for the purposes of computerized statistical analysis. A drug or treatment is deemed 'effective' or even a 'breakthrough' if an arbitrary and quite absurdly small degree of statistical 'improvement' in these pre-defined symptoms is registered. The disorders treated are thought of as 'things in themselves' - disease entities present within the human body or brain of the patient but bearing no specific meaning for the individual human being. The very *selection* of groups of suitable test patients for such studies involves taking a wide range of individuals living in quite different circumstances and, through medical or psychiatric categorizations fitting them to the parameters of the method rather than the other way round. What is ignored in the name of science are all human life factors and feelings which are not subject to quantitative analysis within these parameters.

Paradoxically, despite a relative dearth of controlled clinical studies of its efficacy, much the *same* situation prevails in alternative medicine. For here, no attempt whatsoever is made to distinguish improvements in the patient resulting from a specific mode of physical therapy from (a) the *suggestive* influences of its remedies and ritualized treatment procedures it utilizes, and (b) the therapeutic benefits of the healer-patient *relationship* itself - the healing that comes simply from being fully heard and received as a human being. Nor is there any recognition of the crucial role that might be played by cyclical fluctuations in the severity of a patient's symptoms. For as Freireich showed, many 'alternative' treatments may appear to be effective only because the practitioners are mostly consulted at specific points in a cyclical pattern - either *just before or shortly after* the patient's symptoms reach a peak or a plateau of severity. If, having commenced treatment at this point, the patient goes into a remission or stabilisation phase of their cycle, it is easy for both practitioner and patient to interpret this remission or stabilization as a positive 'result' of the treatment or remedy - which will then immediately take on a positive symbolic and suggestive significance for the patient. If, on the other hand, a practitioner is consulted at the end of a stabilization phase or before a cyclical upturn or peak in the severity of symptoms, the worsening of symptoms following treatment can be interpreted by the practitioner as a necessary part in the healing process initiated by the treatment itself (for example as a phase of 'detoxification'). As if to confirm this hypothesis, the temporary aggravation of the patient's symptoms will indeed be followed by a cyclical phase of stabilization or remission - one which the practitioner can interpret as the treatment finally achieving its desired results. The question is for how long, both in absolute terms and in relation to the overall duration of the course of treatment itself.

The fact that in contrast to many complementary therapies, 'placebo-controlled' studies are central to the testing of orthodox medical treatments should not deceive us however. For the majority of such studies, even where the test results are deemed positive enough for the commercial exploitation of a new drug for example, generally show quite minor differences between patients who received the drug and those on placebo. Above all they completely discount the 'placebo effect' of the drug itself rather than a placebo - the *suggestive significance* of the felt physiological effects it induces, however subtle. At the same time, they generally fail to adequately research adverse reactions of a sort which often more than vitiate a drug's positive results. Short-term reactions, no matter how acute or distressing, are seen as ignorable if they affect only a small minority of patients, and long-term ones rarely even fall within the scope of the research, which is motivated primarily by short- and medium-term commercial prospects. The question *why* a more or less small minority of specific patients suffer side-effects or even die as a result of their treatment or medication, is not only of no intrinsic commercial interest. It is of intrinsically less 'scientific' interest within the parameters of a method in which the *individuality* of the patient as a human being has *already* been eclipsed by some general model of the human body - one in which the felt body and embodied self of the patient have no place.

On the other hand, notwithstanding all the commercial marketing that goes on for 'natural healing' and 'natural' health products, truly natural therapies - rest, sleep and dreams, sensitive and contactful touch massage, and meditative exploration of one's own felt dis-ease - receive virtually no scientific interest or medical respect at all. This is because, if a therapy is to be genuinely natural, it cannot, by its very nature, become either a branded product or the professional and intellectual property of a group of practitioners. Anything worthy of the name 'natural healing' is a property, not of a commercially marketed herb, vitamin or therapy but a capacity for self-healing shared by all human beings and endowed by their body's own knowing - a knowing that requires no medical theory.

The sincere belief on the part of physicians and medical researchers that they *know* the patient's body better than the patients themselves – that they know better than the human being and better than nature, constitutes a type of scientific *hubris* that has already resulted in what Illich aptly describes as medical *nemesis*: a veritable epidemic of medically induced or 'iatrogenic' illness and death on a scale *unparalleled* in human history - the barbarism of 'unscientific' and 'pre-modern' medical treatments notwithstanding. Adverse reactions from legally-prescribed medical drugs, for example, are reported to be the 4th major cause of death in the United States. The problem may be even larger however - for the symptoms of iatrogenic illnesses may not be distinguished by either patient or physician from those of non-iatrogenic disorders.

Medicine is not merely one example amongst others of the application of the modern scientific method. It is itself the paradigm of a rigid scientific world outlook, which seeks causal explanations and technological fixes for every human problem, individual or social, economic or political. A method which takes for granted its own 'objects' of research, and does everything to avoid having to *explore* and *explicate* more deeply the nature of the phenomena that it seeks to explain.

Commenting on Galileo, Heidegger notes that "in the case of the falling apple, Galileo's interest was neither in the apple, nor in the tree from which it fell, but only in the measurable distance of the fall. He therefore supposed a homogeneous space in which a point of mass moves and falls in conformity to law." Such a supposition is the theoretical projection on nature of an unquestioned concept of space, which, in treating all bodies as essentially alike, also treats the human being as a body in space like any other. Questioning the whole relation of theory and experiment in the modern scientific method, Heidegger argues that "the only thing demonstrated is the correspondence of the experimental results to the theory". What is not demonstrated is that this correspondence constitutes genuine knowledge of nature in the way nature itself shows itself outside the framework of our own theoretical representations of it. Instead "the experiment and the result of the experiment do not extend beyond the framework of the theory." That theories are refuted or refined by experiment should not lead us to forget that experiment still remains within the area delimited by theory, and that "what is posited by the theory is the projection of nature according to scientific representations, for instance, those of Galileo". What is decisive in the modern scientific method, and what its experiments seek to refine or refute is "*how* nature is represented, and not *what* nature is".

According to Heidegger this method is no mere 'procedure'. It is "the way and manner in which being, in this case 'nature'... is represented as something standing over and against us, as an object. Neither the ancients nor the medievals represented being as an object. The...objectification of nature is motivated by the idea of representing the processes of nature in such a way that they can be predicted, and therefore controlled." The idea of science as *unmotivated* enquiry into truth is surrendered within the modern scientific method, to a definition of scientific truth as "predictability under controlled conditions" which is entirely *motivated* by the purposes of technological control - but which also gives expression to an abiding fear of Nature in the face of the mystery of Being.

In the modern scientific method the goals of predictability and control go hand in hand with the principle of causal explanation. The search for the causes of an event or phenomenon becomes a universal substitute for understanding its meaning within a larger pattern of significance. Medical science is not merely one application of the causal paradigm. It is the paradigm of a general scientific culture which seeks to locate causes and find 'final solutions' for all human problems rather than exploring their meaning within a larger context. A shy secretary with a bullying and abusive boss restrains her anger but develops instead an 'angry' red skin rash. Going to her GP, the latter seeks its 'causes' in some disorder, whose own 'causes' may or may not be known and form part of a theoretically unlimited chain of causes. What the GP does not see is the significance of the patient's symptoms in the larger context of her life and relationships, her way of being in the world and relating to others.

For all his attachment to the modern scientific world outlook, Freud would not even have dreamt of searching for the 'causes' of a particular dream event or phenomenon in some other event or phenomena occurring *in the same dream* - seeking to explain for example, how a dream monster was 'caused' by a dream thunderstorm. And yet we do something similar whenever we look for the causes of a given phenomenon or event in some other phenomena or event occurring within the same *field or context of emergence*.

The basic 'law' of phenomenological science runs directly counter to the law of causality. It is the understanding that *no* phenomenon or event can be reduced to or explained by other phenomena occurring in the same field or context of emergence. Even in everyday, waking life, we do not isolate a phenomenon such as 'wetness', identify a 'cause' for it, and think to ourselves "the rain caused me to get wet". Rather, what we immediately experience is not an isolated phenomenon such as wetness but a larger holistic event of "getting wet in the rain", or "forgetting my umbrella and getting wet in the rain" or "waking up late, leaving the house in an anxious rush, forgetting my umbrella and getting wet in the rain on the way to an important meeting with my bank manager." In doing so we are not positing an 'initial' cause of our wetness in a hypothetically unending temporal chain of causes and effects. On the contrary, we experience our wetness in a larger temporal context that includes not only significant past events (getting up late) but future ones - that anxiously anticipated meeting with the bank manager. Our immediate experience of the phenomenon of wetness is the immediate experience of an event that is essentially *constituted* by its own larger context of emergence.

Heidegger's basic phenomenological rule - that our "explanation" of a phenomenon can reach only so far as our "explication" of the phenomena to be explained - has a direct bearing on the principle of causal explanation. Our explication of a phenomenon is determined by the way we first of all isolate it within a field or context of appearance. Thus we can isolate the observed production of tear drops, regard them as a phenomenon and then erect the 'scientific' hypothesis that this is the causal result of a person's emotional state. Alternatively, however, instead of reducing the observed phenomenon to a purely physical one occurring in the here and now, we can say that what we immediately observe as a phenomenon is not the production of tear drops but a *person crying*. Rather than attempting to identify the 'causes' of this crying we will then attempt to understand the crying within a larger context. Doing so does not merely allow us to better 'explain' some now already *established* phenomenon. It allows us to *experience* the phenomenon itself in a new way - not simply as "a person crying" but as *this* person crying in *this* particular situation and in *those* particular circumstances that surround it.

We are now in a better position to understand what Heidegger means by the terms "explication" and "explanation", and to suggest what meaning they hold, not just in the context of the physical sciences and their methodology but in the framework of *phenomenological* science and the phenomenological method. From a phenomenological perspective "explication" refers to the "reach" of our initial experience of a phenomenon as an event - the extent to which our experience of this event already embraces its own larger spatio-temporal context of occurrence. It makes a difference, for example, whether we reduce both our experience and our explication of an event to an isolated phenomenon such as 'wetness', or instead experience this phenomenon as part of a larger experiential event of "getting wet in the rain", "forgetting my umbrella and getting wet in the rain" etc.

"Explanation", from a phenomenological perspective, does not mean seeking or finding 'causes', let alone arbitrarily posited 'initial causes' for an arbitrarily isolated phenomenon. It means giving expression to our experience of the phenomenon as part of a larger event *constituted* by its own field or context of occurrence. It must be emphasized that understanding phenomena *contextually* rather than *causally* is by no means the same as hypothesising the existence of multiple causes or causal 'factors'. For though an event may involve multiple phenomena, separated in both time and space, what constitutes the event as an event is that these disparate phenomena form part of a larger pattern of meaning or significance. One phenomenon is not the cause of several others nor are these others multiple causes of the one. Instead, all the identifiable *physical* phenomena that make up the event are the *common* expression of a larger *field* of emergence - 'emergence' being the root meaning of the Greek *'phusis'* from which the terms *physics* and *physical* are derived.

Fundamental science, understood as field-phenomenological science, begins with the recognition that all phenomena arise as events *(Ereignisse)* within a larger field or context of emergence and in this way constitute a self-manifestation *(Er-eignis)* of that field. Any phenomenon arising within a field of emergence is not merely an isolated event or phenomenon occurring within that field. Events of emergence are by nature *field-events*.

Yet field-phenomenological science, like the physics of energetic fields, also admits the reality of multiple fields of emergence. With this goes the recognition that any given phenomenon might be the expression of two or more interrelated or overlapping *event-fields* (for example spatial and temporal fields) or constitute a part of two or more field-events. A phenomenon occurring within the overlap region of two or more interrelated or interacting fields of emergence cannot be said to be 'caused' by other phenomena occurring in these fields, or parallel phenomena occurring as part of the same field-event. Indeed, just as physics now recognizes the existence of 'virtual' phenomena such as 'virtual' particles, so does field-phenomenological science acknowledge the reality of field-events and interactions which do not take the form of physically observable phenomena - but which can nevertheless be experienced. A change in the 'atmosphere' of a social gathering or the 'aura' of a person do not constitute physical observable or measurable phenomena. They nevertheless have reality as field-events.

The aim of field-phenomenological research is to broaden any given 'field' of research in the most literal way possible - by expanding our understanding and very experience of phenomena to embrace the broader *fields* of emergence within which they manifest as field-events. It recognizes that whilst all physical phenomena form part of field-events, not all field-events take the form of observable physical phenomena. This does not mean, however, that such events are inaccessible to direct experience and can only be postulated theoretically or mathematically. For such 'intangible' or 'non-physical' events constitute the very fabric of our everyday subjective experience of the world. That is because 'subjectivity', from a field-phenomenological perspective, is the non-local or field dimension of experience as such - essentially irreducible to any locally experienced phenomena, any localised 'subject' or 'object'.

Field events are accessible to consciousness not as locally observed phenomena but as *felt events* - changes occurring in our own non-local field of awareness and affecting our own *felt body*. The felt body itself has a field character whose volume and dimensions cannot be reduced to those of the physical body. Through it, however, we are linked with all those field-events that constitute the invisible fabric of the physical universe itself. It is meditative feeling cognition, *grounded in the felt body* that constitutes the foundation of phenomenological research - not physical observation or mathematical projection alone. The modern scientific method rests on the unfounded assumption that feeling cognition and felt events cannot be subject to processes of mutual experiential confirmation and validation in the same way as observed physical phenomena or logico-mathematical deductions - even though both empirical observation and the intuitive logic of mathematical reasoning also rest ultimately on consensual 'subjective' validation. This is a method that has no place for the felt body and for feeling cognition - reducing feeling as such to individual 'feelings', seeing the latter only as the private property of localised atomic subjects, and identifying all 'cognitive' functions with the mind or brain alone. In this way, physical science fails to extend its own field models of the physical universe to include an understanding of the field character of our own awareness of that universe, and of our intimately felt bodily connection to the very fields of emergence that are its source.

The starting point of science or any mode of knowledge seeking is, as Heidegger emphasized, not the 'facts' of that science but the adoption by a human being - the scientist - of a specific stance or standpoint, attitude or bearing towards the world. The defining stance of modern science is one of treating the world as something which stands over and against (gegen) an 'independent' subject or observer, and which thereby becomes the bodily object (*Gegen-stand*) of the scientist's own theoretical representations, experimentation and technical manipulations. Heidegger firmly rejected the view that phenomenology was 'anti-scientific'. Rather he rejected the basic stance of modern science as one irreconcilable with the fundamental aims of science *as* science - that of searching for and discerning (*scire*) truth. In its place he suggested a different, more authentically scientific stance: not that of a detached subject standing over and against the world as object but the standpoint of resolutely standing *in* the truth of one's own being-in-the-world - one's own embodied relation to the world and one's own direct bodily awareness of the sense or meaning of phenomena.

Both the *ideal* standards of the modern scientific method and an authentic scientific stance in the Heideggerian sense stand in direct contrast to the stance adopted in everyday life. Making sense of things scientifically means going beyond those shared 'common sense' assumptions and tacit common sense 'understandings' that shape our everyday view of what constitutes 'reality'. The 'sense-making' or 'semiotic' processes of everyday life and language are governed by a number of semiotic codes. It is through these codes that common sense or con-sensual understanding of reality is constituted and protected. Three basic codes can be identified:

1. *A code of discourse* in which we tacitly assume a shared understanding of the meaning or sense of common words and utterances.
2. *A code of conduct* governing everyday worldly practices whereby their own commonly accepted sense or 'rationale' is also tacitly assumed.
3. *A code of communication* that sets boundaries on the legitimate doubt that can be cast on the commonly accepted senses of words and the commonly accepted sense or rationale of worldly practices.

Together, these codes constitute a set of unspoken rules which assume certain agreed *points of departure* for any specific social action or interaction, practice or procedure. *Departing* from these rules or questioning these points of departure is, as Harold Garfinkel's studies showed, guaranteed to arouse bewilderment or indignation.

As an example, we can identify three socially-accepted points of departure for a typical medical consultation:

It is tacitly understood that we all know what 'illness' and 'health' are, that they are opposites, and that 'illness' is something 'bad' and 'health' something 'good'.

It is tacitly understood that the patient arranges the consultation because he is suffering symptoms of a possible 'illness' which he wishes to have identified and which he is therefore prepared to be prescribed treatment for.

It is tacitly understood that the patient will describe their symptoms and that the medical practitioner will then seek to arrive at a medical diagnosis of an illness, and recommend a course of treatment aimed at a 'cure', and based on knowledge of the organic physical 'cause' of that illness.

Should a patient reject any or all of these points of departure, or depart from any of the unspoken rules of interaction they give rise to, he or she will be regarded as disruptive or deviant. This often happens in the case of psychiatric patients who may seek help from a medical practitioner but who may doubt that they are 'ill', doubt that they are in need of 'treatment' or doubt that they're suffering from symptoms with an organic cause.

Scientific sense, in contrast to 'common sense', places, in principle, no boundaries on legitimate doubt or questionability. In practice however, the situation is quite different. For being itself a social practice, modern science is governed by its own codes of discourse, conduct and communication, and by the points of departure implied by these codes.

What have a medical consultation or the nature of therapeutic dialogue to do with the defence of an authentic scientific methodology? Medicine and psychotherapy are areas where the modern scientific and everyday attitudes to sense-making meet. They are also areas in which an authentic scientific stance is *compromised* by a set of pre-established social practices which, being accepted *as a part* of everyday life, are neither socially nor scientifically questioned. The compromising of scientific methodology is particularly prevalent in professional practices such as medicine, and psychotherapy.

A professional practitioner is someone who applies methods derived from an inherited body of scientific knowledge, and hopefully also keeps up to date with new research. A scientist is someone who not only learns how to apply certain methods more effectively but uses their own experience to add to and deepen the body of knowledge which was the source of those methods. Both the scientist and the professional practitioner begin by accepting an inherited body of knowledge on faith. But the professional practitioner who is also a scientist - a knowledge seeker -

goes on to question the limits and explore the gaps in this body of knowledge. There is no reason why an engineer, as a professional practitioner of an applied science, should of necessity also be a research scientist. But the same does not apply to a physician, psychiatrist or psychotherapist. A scientific physician or psychologist is someone motivated and able to learn something more about the human body and human beings from their every bodily encounter with another human being. In the past, every physician was at the same time a scientist, gathering not only new experience but also gaining new scientific insights from that experience. The same was true of psychologists such as Freud. Today, however, we acknowledge entire professions of health 'practitioners' who do not feel any need to be scientists – who apply a general body of knowledge to particular individuals but have no interest in deriving new insights of general validity from their experience of particular patients or clients. Instead they see themselves only as professional practitioners - their sole job being to *incorporate* each new person's experiences into a general body of knowledge, to make sense of it in existing terms and respond to it according to their training. Such a 'know enough already' or 'know it all already' attitude may be 'scientifically' adequate for the job of a professional engineer, who is unlikely to discover new laws of mechanics building a bridge. It is wholly inadequate and inadmissible for a practitioner of the applied human sciences, who will invariably be confronted with scientifically significant differences in each new human being to whom the existing body of scientific knowledge is applied.

Thus the search for a standard and generic medical *diagnosis* replaces the development of new insights from *gnosis* - direct acquaintance with particular patients. The adoption of standard sense-making procedures applies no less in psychotherapy, alternative medicine and complementary health practices as in orthodox medicine and psychiatry. The practitioner seeks merely to identify and remedy a pre-classified 'condition' - whether an organic disorder or childhood disturbance, a chemical imbalance in a person's brain or an 'energy imbalance' in their 'aura', a blocked artery, blocked emotion or a blocked acupunctural 'meridian', a psychological trauma or 'miasm' (homoeopathy).

Of chief concern to the 'professional' is the correct and effective application of a body of knowledge with which to make sense of and respond to the client's emotional signals or bodily symptoms. Of considerably lesser concern is the patient's or client's own *semiotic process* - the way they make sense of and respond to their felt condition and its felt sense or meaning. The client is expected only to *signify* their condition in conventionalized language that can be 'understood' and 'made sense of' by the professional, and to do so in a time-constrained context governed by its own already established semiotic codes, points of departure and routinised or ritualized procedures.

The current one-sided scientific definition of 'semiotics' as the study of signs rather than sense, together with the definition of 'semiosis' as the process of *sign making* rather than *sense-making* fits in well with the semiotic codes governing social and scientific practices in general, which are about 'making the right signs', using the 'right' discourse codes or jargons, and responding 'appropriately' to signs made by others - rather than making deeper sense of those signs. But for this to happen professional practitioners must be able, according to Heidegger, to "glance out beyond their profession and practice and...for once open themselves, let themselves into something entirely different."

The emergence of the modern scientific method shook the foundations and departed from the once universally shared assumptions of the pre-modern religious world view previously dominant in the West. However, an authentic scientific attitude has now been sacrificed to the semiotic codes governing its own institutionalized practice and to the scientific method as this is currently understood - a method largely applied in the service of corporate profit or to sustain the legitimacy of professional bodies. The continuing development of phenomenological science in defence of an authentic scientific stance and an authentically scientific methodology will in turn shake the foundations of the modern scientific method and revolutionise both the theoretical foundations and social practices stemming from that method. It will be grounded in the understanding of both human and natural phenomena as the expressions of fundamental semiotic processes - of *semiosis*.

Not just linguistic signifiers but all phenomena have a semiotic or sign function. But signs do not exist in isolation. The sign function of a word has to do with its place within a larger pattern of linguistic *signification*. The sign function of a phenomenon has to do with its place within a larger pattern of *significance*. A table is not just an extra-linguistic object to which we attach the verbal signifier 'table'. Even without naming it as such, the table already functions as a sign within a larger pattern of significance, being perceived as a place around which we can sit, a platform on which we can eat or write etc. The phenomenon is not merely 'a table' but, for example, the table that someone bought at a bargain price just after getting married or moving house. Similarly, a street is no mere neutral object of perception. What I see of it or do not see of it is determined by its place within a larger pattern of significance. What I see is not 'a street' but *the* street I cross to get into my car or walk down to the local shop.

The semiotic dimension of phenomenology consists in understanding what a phenomenon is in terms of what it means to us - its place within a larger pattern of significance, actual or potential. What both modern science, pre-modern religious world views and 'post-modernism' share in common, however, is a search for an order or pattern of significance to events. Their common point of departure is the assumption of a pre-given order of things - whether divine, natural or purely linguistic or symbolic. In this respect they ignore the very essence of semiosis, which is the process of emergence (*phusis*) of actual patterns of significance from a field of *potential* patterns - the emergence of order from pre-order. Pre-order is not disorder or chaos but consists of potential patterns of significance or signification that are not themselves manifest as actual patterns or phenomena. Indeed the very identification of any actual pattern of significance and its representation in a sign system - linguistic or mathematical patterns of signification - tend to foreclose our awareness of other potential patterns of significance and signification.

Common, everyday sense-making and the consensual reality it assumes, consists of already established patterns of significance represented and reinforced by the accounts we give of them within already established languages or patterns of signification. Scientific sense too, seeks to fit new phenomena into already identified patterns of significance represented in the form of mathematical models or scientific 'laws'. Whether or not new experimental data fit these models is less important than the fact that in common with religion and common sense, science assumes a pre-given order of things that can ultimately be represented in one way or another. New models and the patterns of significance they represent, are created on the basis of earlier ones, and therefore however distinct from the latter, are at the same time inseparable from them and shaped by them. In social-scientific practices such as medicine, we see again the assumption of a pre-given order consisting of already established patterns of significance. Thus a patient's symptoms have meaning only as possible signs of a pre-given and already established disease pattern. Tests are conducted to either confirm or rule out the *actuality* of this possible disease pattern, without any regard to other *potential* patterns of significance unrecognized within the diagnostic framework of medical discourse.

The search for order in science, religion and common sense is self-fulfilling. For any pattern of significance, once identified, limits our awareness of alternate potential patterns and shapes our experience in a way that actively selects out phenomena that do not fit into established patterns or provide signs of other patterns. What Garfinkel called the 'documentary method' is this semiotic process whereby events are interpreted in terms of an already established pattern of significance, and thus provide further 'evidence' of the reality of that pattern. That the perceived pattern of significance itself may be represented in the form of *documents* (for example medical histories or case notes, business reports and legal reports, academic or scientific papers etc) is itself important - for these not only represent perceived commercial, legal, medical or scientific 'realities' according to their own semiotic codes and patterns of signification, but play a powerful role in the way these realities are perceived. Indeed, as documents they form part of the very realities they document. Thus a set of medical test results or a scientific paper does not merely document a specific social practice - that of medical examination or scientific experimentation. As a document it also forms an important part of those practices, laying the basis for further tests or experiments.

The 'hypothesis' of a certain potential pattern of significance in phenomena can be confirmed by experiment or experience. Merely to confirm the phenomenal actuality of a potential pattern of significance however, by no means disproves the reality of other potential patterns, nor does it rule out the existence of alternate, actual patterns. The fact that a vast corpus of sentences, for example, can be shown to share the same syntactic pattern, does not disprove the reality of other potential patterns or the existence of sentences with different syntactic patterns. Similarly, the fact that a person or particle can be shown to exhibit a certain predictable pattern of behaviour proves neither that they do not also exhibit other patterns of behaviour, nor that they do not possess the potential for these other behaviours. In the modern scientific method, it is readily admitted that everything hinges on 'conditions' under which phenomena are observed to follow a predictable pattern, just as in daily life it is readily admitted that everything hinges on the 'situations' in which people behave in certain predictable ways. The question of how conditions or situations are defined, how they can be said to be 'the same' or 'different' is another matter however. Every determination of an experiential situation or set of experimental conditions is already a pre-determination of what counts as a determining 'factor' for the phenomena under investigation.

Dimensions
of Field-Phenomenological Medicine

Field-phenomenological foundations

Both the physical and biological sciences of our day are based on a belief in miracles - the miraculous emergence of *awareness* and aware beings from an otherwise *non-aware* universe of matter and energy - of bodies in space and time. It seeks to explain our *capacity* for conscious awareness through studying particular phenomena within our own *field* of awareness - for example the physical body or brain. The terms 'physical' and 'physics' derive from the Greek verb *phuein* - to 'emerge', 'arise' or 'manifest'. Physics offers explanations of how things emerge or arise but does not begin by recognising them as phenomena emerging or arising within a *field of awareness*. From a phenomenological point of view, the known universe is not merely a universe we happen to be aware of and can therefore attain knowledge of. The universe as we know it is the universe *of* our present human awareness. Deepening and broadening our knowledge of both human and natural phenomena can therefore take two forms - researching and representing relationships between them or deepening and broadening our own *awareness* of them.

The focus of *field-phenomenological* science is not a world of pre-given 'things' independent of our own awareness, but the very nature of those things as phenomena manifesting in a field of awareness. Its basis is a *field-dynamic phenomenology*, one which deals with the *physical* dynamics of phenomena in the root sense of this term - the dynamic process by which phenomena emerge or arise (*phuein*) - not as objects of observation for a localised 'subject' of awareness but as events occurring in a non-localised field of awareness. The observer is but one localised centre or locus of this non-localised field of awareness, which includes both observer and observed. The observed phenomenon gives form to the observer's awareness of the field as a whole. But the awareness that constitutes this field as such is not an awareness *of* any phenomena at all. Within field-dynamic phenomenology, awareness is *not*, as Husserl claimed, essentially awareness *of* something, still less a mental act on the part of a subject or ego which turns these phenomena into 'intentional objects'. Instead any given phenomenon is itself a patterned figuration *of* awareness - one which both gives shape to the source *field* of awareness from which it emerges and *configures* its own awareness of other phenomena within that field. The dynamic relation between *field* and *phenomenon* can be compared to the relation between an ocean and the life forms that emerge within it. Each of these life forms gives form to the life of the ocean as a whole and is in this sense a *self-manifestation* of it. But the very *form* of each of these life-forms also configures their awareness of the ocean as a whole and of all other life forms within it. The shark is aware of the ocean and perceives its other life-forms in a quite different way to the jellyfish. Indeed, what appears to *us* as the form of a shark or jellyfish may bear little comparison to the way the jellyfish perceives the shark and vice versa. As human beings, we are not divinely gifted with a unique figuration or field-pattern of awareness that allows us to perceive the 'true' form of a shark, jellyfish or any other organism. What any organism essentially is, is nothing more or less than an organising *field-pattern of awareness*, one which in-forms its own *patterned field of awareness* and configures its perception of other organisms within that field. The organising field-patterns of awareness that constitute a shark or jellyfish each in-form their awareness both of the ocean as a whole and of other life-forms within it. Each is at the same time the individualised self-manifestation of the life of the ocean as whole.

From a field-phenomenological perspective, since all phenomena are the patterned self-manifestation of source fields of awareness, no phenomenon can ultimately be explained by or reduced to *any other* phenomena manifesting *within* the same field and in-formed by the same field-patterns. Nor can fields of awareness as such be explained by or reduced to the physical phenomena that emerge within them. To do so is comparable to looking for the 'causes' of a dream in the dream, or looking for the causes of a text in that text. Understood phenomenologically, fields of awareness are the *condition* for us becoming aware of any phenomena whatsoever, but are not reducible to or explainable by any phenomena we can observe within them.

The identification of subjectivity with a localized subject or ego is the philosophical reflection of the standard physical scientific model of visual perception. According to this model, seeing is a result of light being reflected off objects in the world and coming to focus in the human eye. This optical focus in the human eye is the analogue of the localized subject or "I". The brain then supposedly interprets signals channeled by the optic nerve and someone produces and projects an 'image' of the object perceived. This physical-scientific model of visual perception is self-contradictory in a double sense. For one thing, it begins by assuming the existence of a pre-given world of physical objects from which light is reflected, and ends up arguing that these objects are in fact effigies - projected mental images produced by the human brain. Secondly it ignores the fact that what we know of the human eye and brain comes from studying them too as objects of visual perception. It rests not only on the assumption that *perceived* objects 'are' as we perceive them to be. It also rests on the assumption that *perceiving objects* i.e. 'organs' of perception such as eye and brain are also pre-given physical objects which appear to us just as they are. There is an inherent paradox in not recognizing that our very knowledge of the body's organs of perception is conditioned, and therefore perhaps limited by our bodily perception of them. The paradox consists in explaining the processes of visual and sensory perception through studying the very products of these processes, for example our visual perception of the human eye and brain.

Physical science starts with the idea of a pre-given world of localised subjects and the objects they perceive in space. The subjects too are perceived as objects (bodies, brains, eyes etc) and the process of perception is explained as a mechanism whereby light from perceived objects impinges and comes to a focus in perceiving objects. From a phenomenological point of view, we do not perceive objects in empty space. Rather space is nothing more or less than the spatial field of awareness itself. Ordinary visual perception can no more be explained by events and interactions occurring within this space or field of awareness than can our visual perception of dream objects be explained by events and interactions occurring in the dream itself. The basic error of the physical-scientific model lies in the attempt to explain phenomena occurring *within* a field of awareness through their 'causal' relations to other phenomena within that field. This is like seeking to find the cause of a particular dream object or event in some other objects or events manifesting within the dream, ignoring the fact that both the caused and the causal object or event are dreamt phenomena - joint manifestations of a singular field of awareness.

The physical-scientific world outlook treats awareness as such as a localised 'epiphenomenon' - a product of physical events and interactions. As a result, it is left with the unanswerable question of how exactly awareness can be generated by these physical phenomena, given its essential and qualitative difference from them. The unanswerable question is ultimately a false and misleading one, for it ignores the fact that physical phenomena are, first and foremost, phenomena emerging or occurring *within* a field of awareness. Physically, perception can be represented as a process in which light reflected off objects in space comes to focus in the human eye. Phenomenologically, the very opposite occurs. The perceptual process is one in which a larger 'peripheral' field of awareness – the light of awareness - comes to a focus as a perceived object 'in' space.

The basic principles of a Fundamental Science as field-phenomenological science - grounded in an understanding of the field character of awareness or subjectivity itself - can be summarized as follows:

Fields of awareness cannot be reduced to or causally explained by the phenomena that manifest within them. We can no more find the 'causes' of illness in the bodily phenomena that emerge within our field of awareness than we can find the causes of 'bad' language or poor sentence construction in a text itself, or the causes of a nightmare in some monster that appears within it.

Phenomena manifesting in a field of awareness cannot be reduced to or causally explained by reference to other phenomena manifesting in the same field. Example: a monster in a nightmare cannot be said to be caused by other objects or events *in* that same nightmare. Similarly, it makes no sense to claim that certain words or sentences in a text are 'caused' by other words and sentences in that text, for the latter too are self-manifestations of a con-textual field of *awareness* linking author and reader.

The words *phenomenon* and *phenomenology* derive from the Greek verb *phainesthai* - to 'shine forth' or 'come to light'. Phenomenological science distinguishes between *physical phenomena* on the one hand and primordial phenomena on the other. A physical phenomenon is an event occurring within a field of awareness (eg. hearing a word spoken) or an object perceived within such a field eg. seeing a word on the page. A primordial phenomenon (what Goethe called an *Urphänomen*) is not something merely present or 'given' in our field of awareness. It is a phenomenon in the *primordial sense* - that which *comes to presence* or 'comes to light' in that field. It must be emphasized that the word 'light' is not used here as a metaphor but in its primordial sense. What we perceive as physical light is something which is itself only visible *in the light* of our own awareness of it. The 'light of awareness' is light in the primordial sense. It is what Heidegger referred to as "the clearing" (*Lichtung*), his term for the open region or "field" (*Feldung*) of awareness which is the condition for anything coming to light as a phenomenon, and which "is not only free for light and darkness, but also for resonance and echo, for sound and the diminishing of sound...the open region for everything that becomes present or absent."

It is in fact modern physics which uses the term 'light' as a metaphor drawn from the realm of our everyday experience of light and darkness, and applied to describe something in no way 'visible' within this realm - for science has long since ceased to regard light as merely the visible part of the electromagnetic spectrum. Instead it now sees the photon as the basic energy 'quantum' or wave-particle mediating *all* electromagnetic interactions. Coming to light (*phainesthai*) has the nature both of physical emergence (*phusis*) and of speech (*logos*). The written or spoken word can be regarded as a physical phenomenon - as ink marks on a page or sound waves traveling through the air. Meanings too, can be turned into objects as if they were just present, pre-given entities. But the word as word - as a primordial phenomenon - can never be reduced to a pre-given object or set of objects. It is not something present but the *coming to presence* of a meaning. To be sure, we can define or describe meanings *as if* they too were pre-given objects. But in this way the process by which meanings *come to light* in language and words *come to mean* what they do will always elude us.

The third basic principle of phenomenological science is that *primordial phenomena cannot be reduced to or explained by physical phenomena.* We do not understand words because we hear them spoken or see them on the page and our brains then 'decode' or 'interpret' them as physical phenomena. We understand words because, as *aware beings,* we already dwell within the *world of meaning* from which they emerge. If I am disturbed by the sounds of loud music being played in the room next door, I am aware of a physical phenomenon, sound vibrations, but I am not actually hearing music. We understand music not because our ears and bodies pick up sound vibrations and audible 'tones' but because we already dwell as aware beings within the world of *feeling tone* from which music emerges. But trying to logically justify the phenomenological standpoint to a scientist or positivist philosopher is a hopeless endeavour - for it is like trying to explain words and music to someone who has no experience of reading or hearing music. We can, by definition offer no physical 'evidence' of primordial phenomena such as meaning, feeling, love etc. The scientist, examining the marks on the page or the oscillations of sound waves in the air will and can find no empirical evidence of an invisible 'world' of meaning or an inaudible world of feeling - any more than they can find empirical evidence of grief in tears. The philosopher will rightly argue that the existence of such worlds cannot be logically proved. Only someone who has already learnt to read or appreciate music to a certain extent will be persuaded of their reality as primordial phenomena.

Principles of field-phenomenological medicine

Biological medicine focuses on illness as a biological phenomenon ie. as a physical phenomenon in the broad sense. Phenomenological medicine is concerned not only with illness as a physical phenomenon – an identifiable symptom or syndrome for example - but with what this symptom or syndrome brings to light. Following the basic principles of field-dynamic phenomenology it does not accept etiologies which seek to explain illness as a physical phenomenon in terms of other physical phenomena which are then treated as its 'causes'. Instead it seeks to understand the patient's awareness of their illness and direct experience of their symptoms in the larger context of the field or 'world' of awareness in which they dwell.

Awareness is intrinsically *relational* - an awareness of ourselves *in relation to* something or someone other than self. A secretary who feels humiliated by her boss, but unable to speak out and confront him develops a visible skin rash on her face and goes to her GP. The physician is not in the least interested in the symptom as a primordial phenomenon - in the humiliation, shame and pregnant anger that the red rash *brings to lig*ht and makes visible - but only in the physical phenomenon. Just as for our scientist and positivist philosopher, there was no proof, empirical or logical that words and sounds point to a world of meaning and feeling, so for the physician the idea that symptoms might have meanings and not just causes is unprovable speculation. His interest is in illness as a physical rather than a primordial phenomenon, in the human body and not in human beings as such, still less in the worlds or fields of awareness in which they dwell; that is to say in the *fields of relatedness* in which they find themselves and comport themselves.

We can study and respond to illness as a physical phenomenon or understand the physical signs of illness themselves in terms of what they bring to light - as primordial phenomenon. Both conventional and alternative medicine focus on the physical *causes and cures* of disease. Neither seek to explore the human being's *awareness* of *dis-ease* and the *meaning* it holds for them in their life. As far as diagnosing the patient's symptoms is concerned, it is as if someone's words would be treated purely as physical phenomena: subject to exacting linguistic, phonological and grammatical analysis without any attempt to hear what they are *saying* through them. We can subject someone's words to detailed phonological, syntactic and even 'semantic' analysis without in any way hearing what the human being is saying through them. Similarly, neither X-rays or blood tests, can tell us anything about a person's awareness of disease, or indeed about their *physiology* in the primordial sense – what emerges or comes to presence (*phusis*) through the speech (*logos*) of the body.

There is today not a single form of medicine, orthodox or alternative, biogenetic or psychoanalytic, Western or Eastern, that does not in one way or another confuse the measurable organic signs of disease with the human being's own felt experience of illness – their *dis-ease*. We can measure a person's heart pressure and pulse. We can diagnose disorders of the heart and circulation. But can we measure heartbreak, heartlessness or 'loss of heart'? The human being's dis-ease, whether in the form of stress or distress, discomfort or pain, anxiety or demoralising incapacity, is not itself anything measurable, whatever its measurable bodily or behavioural signs. The confusion of disease with dis-ease rests, however on a far more fundamental distinction between the physical body and the felt or lived body, the body as a physical phenomena and the body as a primordial phenomenon.

It is this fundamental distinction that Heidegger pointed to through the German words *Körper* and *Leib*. The Leib or lived body is not *only* the so-called 'lived' or 'experienced' body: the body as we are aware of it from within rather than the body perceived from without as a physical object. It is the unified field of our bodily *awareness*, a field that embraces both the 'inner' field of our 'subjective' bodily self-awareness with the 'outer' field of our own 'objective' sensory awareness of the world and other bodies within it. It is for this reason that Heidegger could declare that: "The lived body (*Leib*) is certainly no thing, no corpus (*Körper*), but every body; in other words the body as *Leib* is always my body."

By this he meant that our awareness of our own bodies and of other bodies in our environment are not separate. For one thing, our awareness of other bodies in our outer physical environment, whether those of objects or people, co-constitutes our inner awareness of our own physical bodies and vice versa. In the neighbourhood of extremely tall, large or heavy persons our own bodies feel shorter, smaller or lighter for example. The contrast between the anorexic's experience of their own bodies as gross or fat and other people's perception of them as waif-like and starved cannot be put down to the 'body image' of the former.

Bodily self-image has to do with how we imagine ourselves to appear to others from without. What the anorexic is describing is not a mental image of their own physical body as this appears from without but a sense of their own lived or felt body - the body as they experience it from within. The lived body, as Heidegger pointed out, is not essentially bounded by the measurable dimensions of the physical body. We can feel fatter or lighter, taller or shorter, without physically fattening or lightening, and without our measurable height changing in any degree at all. And "When I direct someone towards a windowsill with a gesture of my right hand, my bodily existence as a human being does not end at the tip of my index finger. While perceiving the windowsill....I extend myself bodily far beyond this fingertip to that windowsill. In fact, bodily I reach out even further than this to touch all the phenomena, present or merely visualised, represented ones."

Heidegger's conclusion is a radical one "The boundary of the lived body is the horizon of being in which I dwell." As a larger body or unified *field of* awareness, it embraces both our experience of ourselves and our experience of others and otherness, including both our 'proprioception' of our own bodies and our perceptual awareness of other bodies around us. Understood phenomenologically, both our experience of ourselves *as* localized subjects *and* the objects that we perceive around us are inseparable aspects of a singular field of awareness. It is this *larger body or field of awareness* that we are in the habit of thinking of merely as the pre-given physical 'space' in which our bodies are located, a space which, according to the scientific model, somehow happens to contain both perceived objects and subjects capable of perceiving them and the space in which they exist. A space which happens to contain physical *objects* of a special and miraculous sort - bodies with eyes and brains which miraculously generate subjective awareness of themselves and mysteriously 'contain' a localised subject which projects mental images of space and of objects *into* the very space in which it is supposedly located *as* an object in the first place.

The unrecognized and unresolved paradoxes of this model make it rather unconvincing, to say the least, and Heidegger was not averse to pointing out the double standards involved in applying it.

"When it is claimed that brain research is a scientific foundation for our understanding of human beings, the claim implies that the true and real relationship of one human being to another is an interaction of brain processes, and that in brain research itself, nothing else is happening but that one brain is in some way 'informing' another. Then, for example, the statue of a god in the Akropolis museum, viewed during the term break, that is to say outside the research work, is in reality and truth nothing but the meeting of a brain process in the observer with the product of a brain process, the statue exhibited. Reassuring us, during the holidays, that this is not what is really implied, means living with a certain double or triple accounting that clearly doesn't rest easily with the much faulted rigour of science."

Ontological dimensions
of field-phenomenological medicine

The term 'ontology' derives from the Greek *onto*s – 'being'. The ontological foundation of biological medicine is the reduction of the human *being* to the human body and its biological organs. The basis of human existence and experience, as experienced in the everyday process of *living*, is sought in a purely biological understanding of 'life'. In the topsy-turvy world of medical science it is not human beings that think and feel but their brains which 'produce' thoughts and feelings, 'store' memories etc. and in the process constitute the human being as a being. I term this reductionistic position 'bio-ontology'. Heidegger questioned its basic metaphysical assumptions, arguing instead that the human being cannot be reduced to the human body. On the contrary, the human body and its organic functions can only be understood as an *embodiment* of the intrinsic potentials and capacities of the human *being*. Heidegger often remarked that our understanding of truth depends most essentially on correctly appreciating the obvious. The obvious, in this context, is that it is not ears that listen and hear, eyes that look and see, or *brains* that think but *beings*.

Bodily organs such as the human eye do indeed have *functions* in the same way that tools or instruments such as pens and computers do. The function of a pen is to serve as an instrument of writing - it is something to write with. But however sophisticated its functional design and operation, no pen is *capable* of writing. And seeing and hearing, like writing are essentially *capacities* not functions. As beings we possess a capacity for writing whether or not writing instruments are available, and this capacity belonged to us as a potential of our being even before such instruments were invented. As a functional instrument (Greek *organon*) a bodily organ is the *embodiment* of a *capacity* belonging to the human being - not the basis of those capacities. That is why the very development of our bodily organs depends on the exercise of these capacities. We learn to write, drive or swim *by* writing, driving and swimming. In the process of exercising these capacities - in however primitive a way at first - our brain functioning is itself stimulated, transformed and developed. We do not first alter our brain's neurological functioning and then somehow find ourselves able to exercise a capacity. According to Heidegger "..we cannot say that the organ has capacities, but must say that the capacity has organs." The organ does not 'posses' a capacity but is "in the possession of a capacity" - subservient to it in the same way that the pen is subservient to our capacity to write. For Heidegger life itself is essentially *capability* (*Fähigkeit*). "This capability, articulating itself into capacities creating organs characterizes the organism as such." "It is not the organ which has a capacity but the organism which has capacities."

Heidegger goes even further than this however, suggesting that the very 'organismic' capacities embodied in our organs and their functions are not essentially biological - rooted in our body's genes - but rather ontological, having to do with intrinsic potentials of the human being?

"*We* hear, not the ear...Of course we hear a Bach fugue with our ears, but if we leave what is heard only at this, with what strikes the tympanum as sound waves, then we can never hear a Bach fugue...if *we* hear, something is not simply added to what the ear picks up; rather what the ear perceives and how it perceives will already be attuned (*gestimmt*) and determined (*bestimmt*) by what *we* hear, be this only that we hear the titmouse and the robin and the lark...(O)ur hearing organs...are never the sufficient condition for our hearing, for that hearing which accords and affords us whatever there really is to hear."

"The same holds true for our eyes and vision. If human vision remains confined to what is piped in as sensations through the eye to the retina, then, for instance, the Greeks would never have been able to see Apollo in a statue of a young man...."

Damage to functional organs can itself be the result of inhibition placed on the exercise and embodiment of capacities. An infant with an infection in one eye had a patch placed on the eye for a considerable period during its treatment. When the infection had disappeared and the patch was removed it was found that the child was no longer able to see through this eye. The medical explanation of this phenomenon was that the patch has been placed on the eye at a critical time in the child's neurological development. Lacking visual stimuli, the necessary nerve pathways were not formed for this eye. Put in other words, the patch prevented the child from exercising its *capacity* to see through this eye - with the result that an organic, neurological impairment in its *functioning* resulted. The capacity itself, however, involves far more than simply a functional receptivity of the eye to visual stimuli and their translation into nerve impulses transmitted to the brain. Just as a pen cannot write, nor does the eye or brain itself possess a capacity to see. That capacity is exercised by an aware being not a bodily organ.

Metaphorical dimensions
of field-phenomenological medicine

For Heidegger, thinking itself "is a listening that brings something in view" - that enables us to *see*. But he firmly rejected the view that such 'insight' was a type of 'seeing' only in a *metaphorical* sense. "If we take thinking to be a sort of hearing and seeing, then sensible hearing and seeing is taken up and over into the realm of nonsensory perception…In Greek such a transposing is called *metaphorein*. The language of scholars names such a carrying-over "metaphor". So thinking may be called a hearing and a listening, a viewing and a bringing into view, only in a metaphorical sense. Who says "may" here? Those who assert that hearing with the ears and seeing with the eyes is genuine hearing and seeing."

When we 'see' that somebody is unhappy or tense, or 'hear' frustration in their tone of voice this is not a deduction made from some sort of quasi-clinical observation. Similarly, when our impression of somebody is that they look or sound 'unwell' we are not, like the physician, medically interpreting certain overt diagnostic 'signs'. What Heidegger refers to as "genuine" seeing or hearing is not, in the first place, a seeing or hearing which has as its object something or 'some-body' in the literal sense, but rather 'some-one' - a *being* and not a body in space and time.

What I have termed the 'phenomenal' body as opposed to the physical body is precisely that body with which we directly see and hear, sense and feel, touch and move other *beings*, doing so quite independently of physical sight and hearing, touch and movement. When we speak of being close to someone, being touched by their words or moved by their suffering it is not physical intimacy, touch or movement we are referring to. Nor however, is our reference to closeness, touch and movement merely a metaphorical way of describing in physical terms something psychical. Rather the converse - moving closer to someone physically or touching them in an intimate way is itself a form of metaphorical action - a way of 'bearing across' (*metaphorein*) our closeness to them as beings.

Bodily intimacy, intercourse and reproduction, far from being the biological foundation of human behaviour are themselves the expression of an ontological capacity for intimacy with other human *beings*. When human beings engage in sexual intercourse their body temperature rises like that of other animals. But the *warmth* they feel for one another as beings is not a measurable physical phenomenon but a primordial one, independent of its expression in bodily warmth and temperature. The term 'onto-biology' refers to an ontological understanding of biological functions of the sort that Heidegger indicated. This is not the same thing as a psychological or psychoanalytic understanding of such functions. When someone speaks of feeling 'stifled' or of having no 'room to breathe' this is not usually meant in a literal sense, but nor are they merely describing an emotional or 'psychological' state using a respiratory metaphor. But if someone's breathes more freely as a result of feeling their 'spirits' lift, their bodily breathing does indeed serve as a living, *biological metaphor* of their state of being. Respiration is not merely a biological function but the embodiment of a primordial organismic capacity of our being - the capacity to engage in a rhythmic exchange with the essential 'atmosphere' of our life-world, 'breathing in' our *awareness* of it, drawing inspiration and meaning from it, and in turn allowing our *awareness* to flow out into it and find meaning within it. A person can jog or exercise, or practice Yogic breathing exercises for hours, days or years without it significantly affecting their *fundamental* respiration - without it bringing new sources of spiritual meaning and inspiration into their lives. But a person can be neither spiritually inspired nor dispirited without it being instantaneously embodied in their physical breathing.

At what point does the air we inhale become a part of us? At what point does our exhaled air cease, not only to be a part of our bodies but a part of us? Whether we draw into our awareness a 'breathtaking' landscape or an 'idea', we feel moved to inhale and then exhale deeply. Why? Because breathing is the embodiment of our primordial capacity to fully take into *ourselves* our awareness of something *other than self*, and in turn allow it to freely flow out into the atmosphere or field of awareness linking us with it. The words 'respiration', 'inspiration', 'aspiration' etc. come from the Latin *spirare* - to breathe - just as the Greek word *psyche* originally meant the 'breath' that vitalised an otherwise lifeless corpse (*soma*). To speak in a modern way of the 'psychosomatic' dimension of breathing disorders such as asthma, to either claim or dispute their 'psychogenic' causation therefore misses the point. It ignores the question of what breathing as such fundamentally *is* - not as an organic function of our body but as an organismic capacity of our being. Changes in the pattern and flow of our bodily breathing embody differently patterned flows of awareness. As such they may also provide the medium by which our *relationship* as beings to particular phenomena first *comes to presence* in our field of awareness.

Field-phenomenological medicine identifies the human *organism* neither with the physical body or *soma* nor with the *psyche* understood in the traditional sense - as a localized subjectivity bounded and contained by the physical body.

Instead it understands the organism as the dynamic boundary between the two fields of awareness that constitute our larger body of awareness or felt body - an 'inner' field awareness of our own bodies and 'outer' field awareness embracing other bodies in our sensory environment. The organism as such is the dynamic boundary state that both distinguishes and unites these two fields. As such it is also the dynamic interface between what we experience as 'self' and that which we experience as other-than-self, uniting our self-awareness with our awareness of others and otherness. Self-awareness is also an awareness of ourselves *in relation* to something or someone other-than-self. Indeed it is co-constituted by that very relation. Our self-experience is always inseparable from an experience of others and otherness. The "I" that I experience in the context of one relationship or activity is not identical to that which I experience in another. The "I" experienced in a professional role is not the same "I" experienced in a domestic context or engaged in a pleasurable recreation. When we feel ill, we do not 'feel ourselves', our bodies or minds feel foreign or alien to us in some way. This 'not feeling ourselves' however, is always the expression of change in our *felt relation* to something or someone other-than-self.

Historically, medicine has always interpreted this relationship in an essentially paranoid way. The change in our bodily self-awareness and the sense of foreignness that characterize the felt experience of illness have been represented as the work of a foreign entity – whether a malignant spirit or a foreign body such as a virus or cancer cell. Immunology is founded less on biological fact than on conceptual metaphor – an empirically and biologically highly questionable distinction between so-called 'self' and 'non-self' cells. It is dominated by the military metaphor of the body as a battlefield for a war against foreign 'non-self' cells and organisms, just as medical discourse as a whole is dominated by the metaphor of war against illness as such. Just how pervasive this metaphor is, not just in everyday discourse but in biology itself, can be seen from the language used in the following, quite orthodox accounts of immune functioning. "[W]hen immune *defenders* encounter cells or organisms carrying molecules that say 'foreign', the immune *troops* move quickly to eliminate the *intruders*."

"The immune system *stockpiles* a tremendous *arsenal* of cells. Some *staff* the general *defenses*, while others are trained on highly specific *targets*." {author's italics}

The military metaphor extends beyond immunology and represents the all-embracing metaphor of modern medicine. The metaphor is rigorously defended under the banner of medical 'science' even though it is the foundational metaphor *of* this science, the basic metaphorical framework determining the medical interpretation of empirical data and the scientific representation of biological 'fact'. Behind it is the questionable concept of an *immune self*, constituted by a genetically-programmed biological identity. This concept can be understood as a projection of the traditional metaphysical notion of the subject - the Cartesian ego - on the human body. The root meaning of 'self' is 'sameness'. Biologically, the body is in fact never *the same* from one moment to the next. It constantly recreates itself and does so precisely through the incorporation and assimilation of previously 'foreign', 'non-self' substances - air, water, nutrients etc. Our felt, bodily self is also not a fixed identity - it too recreates itself constantly by assimilating and incorporating our experience of others and otherness.

The human organism is our felt, bodily sense of self - a sense of self that is ever-changing, forever and continuously altered by our felt relation to others and otherness. The *ego* on the other hand is a mental identity 'immunised' from its experience. It is the self represented by the linguistic subject – the word "I". When we say "I feel cold" or "I feel hot" we imply that the "I" is the same "I" in both cases, a subject *immune* from its predicates, a subject whose *identity* is never altered by its own verbs and objects, actions and experiences. The ego uses language to identify a feeling as one of "coldness" or "heat", "joy" or "sadness", and to identify 'reasons' why it should be feeling one way or the other. The organism - our felt, bodily sense of self - is fully identified *with* what it feels. It *is* the feeling of coldness or heat, joy or sadness – even if, as is often the case, it has unlike the ego no words to label, represent and objectify the feeling in question.

Medical immunology and the immune self it postulates is an ideologically-shaped representation of and response to the *dis-ease* experienced by the *ego* when its own identity is disturbed by an organismic state - an alteration in the individual's felt, bodily sense of self. Organismic states are in turn the expression of an individual's *felt relation* to something or someone in their outer field of awareness. But just as 'nature abhors a vacuum', so the organism abhors an absence. Life frustrations, deprivations, disappointments, losses and bereavements all represent an experience of absence which the organism can only register to the ego as the positive presence of a particular feeling, albeit a so-called 'negative' feeling such as grief, unhappiness or pain. Actually, such 'negative' feelings are feelings *negated* by the ego, which, unlike the organism seeks to immunise itself from feeling as such.

Whereas the organismic self is the *felt self* - identified *with* what it feels - the ego is the 'immune self' - the part of us that does not allow *what* we feel to alter our identity and transform our sense of *who* we are. The ego has 'feelings' (plural noun). The human organism is like the hand with which we *feel* (verb). If we feel someone's face with our hand, what it feels like to our touch, the 'feeling' (noun) that we have of it, depends on the way we touch it, the way we 'feel' it (verb). For the human being 'feeling' is an activity and not merely a state. And it is we who feel, not our hands. We feel out other beings, sensing their presence or absence, nearness or distance, approach or withdrawal, openness or closedness, weight or lightness of being, and this *feeling out* constitutes our felt body as a 'field' or 'feel-d' of awareness. In feeling we are invariably touched and transformed *by* what we touch and feel. The organism is our felt, bodily sense of self, a bodily self that, unlike the 'immune self' is never the 'same'.

Diagnostic dimensions
of field-phenomenological medicine

An elderly woman whose husband Harry has recently died from a heart attack finds herself suffering chest pains at night and goes to see her GP. The physician's only interest in her symptoms is as signs of a possible organic disorder which might be 'causing' them. He sends her to a consultant to test for possible heart conditions. Proving inconclusive, the consultant ends up diagnosing mild angina, and prescribes tablets. These in turn prove to have little effect on the patient's symptoms. On visiting her GP a second time however, the latter recalls her recent bereavement and, as a result, begins to read the somatic 'text' of her symptoms in a different way, understanding them in the life *context* of her loss and the pain it be may be causing her. Rather than seeking a purely medical diagnosis of the patient's symptoms he himself *listens* to his patient in a genuinely *patien*t way. Suddenly an insight flashes through his mind. He 'sees' that she may be suffering from a doubly broken heart "the one that killed Harry, and the one you're left alive with, that hurts when you're most alone in the middle of the night...the broken heart that gave up and the one has to carry on painfully." This *heartfelt* hearing of the patient and the *heart-to-heart* talk that ensue are the first time anyone has ever *acknowledged* the pain of her grief. It gives her the *strength of heart* to acknowledge and bear it in a new way. Her symptoms disappear.

This case history, which is cited by Dr David Zigmond in an article on different modes of patient-physician communication, goes to the heart of the contrast between medical diagnosis and fundamental diagnosis. The term 'diagnosis' means 'through knowing' (*dia-gnosis*). *Gnosis* derives from the Greek *gignostikein* - to 'know' in the sense of being familiar or intimate with. *Gnosis* is not knowledge *of* or *about* something, but the sort of knowing we refer to when we speak of knowing someone well or intimately. The relation that distinguishes this type of knowing is one in which, as Heidegger put it "*we ourselves* are related and in which the relation *vibrates* through our basic comportment." Medical knowledge, like other forms of scientific knowledge, including psychology, is knowledge of or about. It represents the outer relationships *between* things or between people as if these were quite independent of our inner relation to them - our inner bearing towards them.

The change in the GP's relationship to the patient in the second consultation was crucial. Rather than simply bringing to bear his medical-biological knowledge of the heart, he had the patience to *bear with* his patient - to acknowledge her heartbreak and bear it with her in a heartfelt way. As a result she herself, no longer felt herself so painfully alone in bearing it, and was able as a result, to find a new bearing towards the loss that occasioned it. The paradox is, that despite the inconclusiveness of the medical tests, without adopting this bearing the patient might well have gone on to *bear and body* the pain of her lonely grief through increasingly acute symptoms, using them to feel and communicate it indirectly through a type of 'organ speech'. The GP's new bearing was preventative in the deepest sense, forestalling a process whereby this patient might well have ended up as a genuine 'heart case' requiring medical intervention, or a 'heart sink' case in which no conclusive, measurable signs could be found of any organic disorder. When doctors speak of the 'heart-sink' patient perhaps all that is referred to is the type of patient that *all too clearly* needs this type of fundamental or 'deep' diagnosis, rather than fruitless attempts to diagnose their symptoms in the ordinary way ie, to hear, see and respond to their inner *dis-ease* rather than seeking its causes in a medically labeled disease or disorder.

The focus of biological medicine is certainly not the felt or lived body but rather the *clinical body* - the human body as represented in the body of medical knowledge *about* it that provides the foundation of medical training. The gaze of the physician is a *clinical gaze*, one which turns the body into an object of medical-scientific examination and clinical testing. At its heart is a fundamental separation between the human body and the human being, between biological life processes and the everyday life of the individual, a separation that further distances the patient as a human being from their own body and turns their dis-ease into an impersonal thing - an "It". Medical treatment is seen as identifying and

57

eliminating this "It" - to make "It" go away, or to make "It" better. The physician is not trained to apply a *phenomenological gaze* - to see what specific physical symptoms *bring to light* as phenomena - but rather seeks physical causes for them. His interest is not in the patient's felt *dis-ease* but only its measurable physical signs. The fact is, however, that the patient's dis-ease, distress or discomfort is not itself essentially measurable. The sort of space that 'pain' occupies is not a physical space. The *inwardness* of dis-ease is comparable to the inwardness of the word. It is a *non-spatial* interiority that 'internal medicine' can find no evidence of, no more than it can find evidence of someone's heartbreak or loss of heart by prizing open their chest in surgery. The case described by Zigmond is a pertinent one, given Heidegger's comments on the immeasurability of grief: "How does one measure grief? Obviously we cannot measure it at all. Why not? Were we to apply a method of measurement to grief, this would go against the meaning of grief and we would rule out in advance the grief as grief." Nor can one measure tears, for "when one measures one measures at best a fluid and its drops but not tears." More than once Heidegger approvingly cites Aristotle's remark that "...it is uneducated not to have an eye for when it is necessary to look for a proof and when this is not necessary." Seeking evidence of organic disorder through clinical testing and physical measurements of one sort or another is one thing - though it tells us nothing of what this disorder reveals as a primordial phenomenon, the dis-ease it embodies and brings to light. Seeking evidence or proof of psychiatric disorders through questionnaires or brain scans is 'uneducated' in just the way that Aristotle suggests. For it is rather like needing to prove someone's unhappiness by asking them how often they cry, by looking for 'evidence' in the form of tears or tear stains, or worse still, seeking a reliable 'scientific' index of their unhappiness by weighing their teardrops.

Pathosophical dimensions
of field-phenomenological medicine

"Feeling is the very state, open to itself, in which we stand related to things, to ourselves, and to the people around us."
(Heidegger).

The term 'pathosophy' was coined by Viktor von Weizsäcker, the first scientist and physician to attempt the creation of a 'medicine beyond medicine' - a comprehensive new model of health and illness based both on philosophy and on psychoanalytic depth-psychology. He understood illness as one expression of the 'pathic', defined as "the essential suffering of a person that is related to that which they lack and that towards which they are aiming." The literal Greek meaning of 'pathosophy' is 'the wisdom of suffering' or 'the wisdom of feeling'. The traditional aim of medicine has always been the alleviation or elimination of the suffering experienced by the sick person, and with it the diminution of any intense feelings, fears or anxieties accompanying or amplified by their illness. At the heart of almost all forms of medicine is the assumption that illness and suffering are not only undesirable in themselves but lacking in any intrinsic *meaning*. The practice of medicine is founded on the medicalisation and medication of disease, which is reduced to some form of diagnosable mental or physical 'pathology' and not in any way seen as a meaningful expression or embodiment of the *pathic*. The suffering of the human being is seen as an expression of their medical condition. The medical condition is never seen primarily as an expression of an individual's problems but as the problem itself. There is no question of seeing their bodily or behavioural 'pathology' as the meaningful embodiment and expression of the pathic - of a *felt dis-ease*. For to do so would surely be tantamount to 'blaming the patient for the illness'. But behind this accusation, so often levelled against those who question the accepted wisdom of the medical establishment, lies one of the most concealed and yet basic assumptions of medicine in all its forms - the assumption that illness and suffering are something *blameworthy* and therefore 'bad' in the first place, something for which a cause or scapegoat must be found.

Many thinkers have questioned this assumption. Balint argued that "Patients turn their problems into illnesses, and...the physician's job is to turn them back into problems." Groddek saw the meaning of illness as a warning: "Do not continue living as you intend to". Others have gone on to argue that not only is illness a warning sign but that successful 'treatment' or 'cure' is equivalent to simply disabling or destroying the warning light itself. Psychiatric treatment through neuroleptic drugs is a rather literal case in point. For these work precisely by diminishing brain functioning and in the long term producing chronic brain damage. Indeed the very term 'neuroleptic' refers to the way these drugs simulate the effects of brain disease or brain damage. As far as the toxicity effects of medical treatment in general are concerned, the facts speak for themselves - it is the single largest *medical* cause of death after heart disease, stroke, cancer and AIDS. As for the benefits we all *assume* modern medicine to have brought and to be furthering through its scientific development, the empirical data suggests otherwise. By the time antibiotics began to be used widely the major infectious diseases had already gone through their most dramatic decline, attributed primarily to better housing and nutrition. Today the life-expectancy of untreated cancer patients is significantly higher than that of those treated with chemo- and radiotherapy. There is no statistical evidence for the efficacy of (expensive) intensive care units. "Neither the proportion of doctors in a population nor the clinical tools at their disposal nor the number of hospital beds is a causal factor in the striking changes in overall patterns of disease." (Illich) Nor have they contributed to improvement in life-expectancy. If anything, quite the opposite. For, the vast sums of money spent on medical care in developed countries, and, increasingly by the developing ones has deprived the latter of crucial resources for dealing with poverty, malnutrition and starvation, the latter being still the single largest cause of death in the world.

"Health and suffering as experienced sensations are phenomena that distinguish men from beasts. Only storybook lions are said to suffer..." (Illich). In the past, spiritual meaning was attached to illness, and different cultures each had their own rituals for the vital expression and communication of human suffering. Today's culture, on the other hand, regards the medicalisation and medication of suffering as the only *rational* response to it, and perceives the rejection of medical help as vain masochism. "Blaming the patient" means making them responsible *for* their suffering. Medicine does the opposite. It deprives human beings not only of their responsibility for suffering but 'response-ability' to it - their ability to *respond* to their own felt dis-ease and thereby experience their suffering not as passive surrender to fate but as a meaningful and responsible *activity*. Children tend to actively express and embody their moods, their sense of ease or dis-ease, communicating it through their bodily countenance and demeanour. Parents however, often react harshly to any attempt on the part of the child to actively communicate their suffering in a bodily or behavioural way - telling the child, for example, not to sulk or brood, not to make a long face. The child is taught that suffering is something to be privatised and masked or else communicated only in a verbal way - that it must on no account be actively *bodied.*

"Every feeling is an embodiment attuned in this or that way, a mood that embodies in this or that way." (Heidegger). Actively *bodying* feelings is not to be confused with what psychoanalysts call 'acting out'. 'Acting out' is actually 'reacting out' - a reactive behavioural response *to* a particular feeling which prevents us from having to *feel* that feeling in a more direct bodily way and to find a bearing that allows us to bear or contain it. Acting out feelings through our behaviour is essentially a *flight* from feeling those feelings, albeit one which may take the form of a *fight* response which serves to discharge and evacuate the feeling. To *body* a feeling or attunement means simply to allow ourselves to feel that feeling in a bodily way, and to let it take shape in a bodily way - to express itself as a bodily demeanour or comportment. This is quite different from just representing and relaying what we feel in words or suppressing it in silence. Nor is it the same as a reactive response to what we feel which takes the form of 'neurotic' patterns of verbal or non-verbal behaviour. To body a feeling is to let it be what it essentially is - "an embodiment attuned in this or that way, a mood that embodies in this or that way". The phenomenological, ontological and medical significance of this understanding of *feeling* and their intrinsic relationship to bodyhood cannot be overestimated. For as Heidegger himself suggested:

"We know by now a great deal - almost more than we can encompass - about what we call the body, without having seriously thought about what *bodying* is. It is something more and different from merely 'carrying a body around with one'." "As simple and obscure as that which we know as gravitation is, gravity and the falling of bodies, the *bodying* of a living being is just as simple and just as obscure." "The *bodying* of life is nothing separate by itself, encapsulated in the 'physical mass' in which the body can appear to us..."

Psychosomatic dimensions of field-phenomenological medicine

Heidegger asks "To what do tears belong? Are they something somatic or something psychic?" His answer: "Neither one nor the other." That is because the very question assumes the existence of 'psyche' and 'soma', 'soul' and 'body' as separate pre-given entities whose relation and interaction then needs to be explained or accounted for.

The body itself is understood as a 'body-thing' rather than as the bodying of a being. From an onto-phenomenological perspective, tears are neither psychic nor somatic but weeping is quite simply one mode of bodying - the embodiment of a state of being. In psychoanalytic literature, however, the term 'bodying' (equivalent to the German *leiben*) does not exist. In its place is the term 'somatisation'. The psychoanalytic explanation of the so-called 'psychosomatic' dimension of illness is that the *pathic* takes the form of a somatic *pathology* through the process of *somatisation*. Feelings not given form as verbal symbols will be experienced instead as somatic states and sensations and find expression in somatic symptoms and disorders. The tendency to somatise feelings results from an inability to cognitively 'process' them – to mentally represent what one is feeling and relay it in words. The term *alexithymia* has been coined to denote this deficiency in the cognitive processing of one's emotional life. This psychoanalytic model is phenomenologically questionable for a number of reasons. To begin with one might ask how it is possible for an individual to *mind* their own feelings - to acknowledge them in words or 'process' them cognitively - without first feeling and giving form to those feelings in some bodily way, without bodying them? The model assumes we begin with two separate things - a *disembodied* and *disarticulated* emotion on the one hand and its somatic or verbal expression on the other. The model suggests that what is experienced by the *alexithymic* individual only as a bodily sensation is really an emotion in disguise. If so, what sort of reality does this emotion have, and what sort of psychic space does it occupy *prior* to the cognitive processing necessary to acknowledge it as an emotion?

This is an important question because the model does imply that emotions are not merely the result of cognitive processing and verbal labeling of feelings but some sort of pre-given entity – internal psychical objects comparable to external physical objects.

In contrast Heidegger understands feelings not as 'internal objects' or labelled 'emotions' but as *Stimmungen*. These are 'moods', 'attunements' or 'feeling tones' which permeate and colour our awareness of both ourselves and our world, and allow our felt relation to things and people to *resonate* within us. Unlike nameable emotions, such primary feeling tones cannot, according to Heidegger, be 'ascertained' ie. identified and represented in thought. In this they are comparable to musical tones and chords, for though they may evoke nameable emotions in themselves they defy emotional labeling. Independently of any processes of 'somatisation', emotions are already, and in themselves, specific *embodiments* of feeling tone. In the *Zollikon Seminars* Heidegger asks at one point whether a phenomenon such as *blushing* is to be regarded as the psychological experience of a somatic state or the somatic expression of a psychological state – for example an emotion such as embarrassment or shame. In doing so he points to something essential to an understanding of feeling that transcends the mind/body, psyche/soma distinction. The question he poses rhetorically is unanswerable. This is not because of any lack of empirical evidence - for what sort of evidence could offer a definitive answer - but because of the very terms in which it is posed. We cannot therefore, simply rest content with regarding phenomena such as blushing as the somatic expression of emotions such as shame or embarrassment. Nor is it convincing to suggest that the blushing is merely a pre-programmed 'physiological' response that somehow generates or happens to be accompanied by a psychical awareness of such emotions. We can look at such phenomena as blushing or going red with anger in a different way however, seeing *both* the 'somatic' phenomena and the *emotions* that accompany them as ways of bodying a specific feeling tone - a *felt relation* to something or someone that cannot be reduced either to a programmed physiological response or pre-given emotion.

Thus emotions such as 'anger', 'shame' or 'embarrassment' for example are not internal psychical objects or states that exist *prior* to their verbal or physical expression. They are different possible ways of experiencing the same felt relation to something or someone, all of which have in common a certain outward movement or *e-motion*, one which has the specific character of bringing our felt awareness of this relation *to the surface*, not only psychically but also somatically, through the reddening of our faces. Such basic movements or dynamics of *awareness* (establishing a surface boundary, bringing awareness to this surface, expanding or contracting a bounded field of awareness, withdrawing awareness from a surface and 'going into oneself' etc.) are natural ways in which *feeling tones,* as felt relationships to something or someone other than self, *body* themselves. It is not some mentally unacknowledged emotion such as 'grief' but the *tears that are not shed in grief, the loss that is not bodied in tears* which then finds expression in either psychological disturbance or somatic symptoms. We can understand why it is therefore, that the medications used to treat certain conditions suspected of having a 'psychosomatic' dimension (asthma for example) tend to stimulate the very physiological processes that accompany specific psychological *emotions* such as anger. Through purely chemical means they bring about the somatic embodiment of a *motion* that the individual is otherwise incapable of *letting be* and *freely body*ing.

In his essay on "The Essence and Concept of Phusis" Heidegger discusses Aristotle's account of a living being as one whose *movedness* has its order and origin within itself. The term 'movedness' does not refer merely to motion in space but to change and transformation of any sort. The essential character of this movedness is a self-unfolding, which, like that of the plant is at the same time a rooting or grounding movement of 'going-back-into-itself'. Movement as such is something which "has itself within its own end". Rest is not merely the opposite of movement or its mere cessation, but its consummation - the end from which it originates and orders it from within as its essential direction or *telos*. The ceaseless and apparently restless motion that makes up the physiological life of the organism, is at the same time a constant coming to rest - the stabilization of an inner order and organization (*logos*) that manifests (*phusis*) as the bodily form of the organism (morphe). The 'physiology' of a living being is essentially a movedness that bodies and comes to rest in this bodying, not only unfolding from within itself but also, and at the same, constantly going back into itself.

These two basic movements - the movement out of self-unfolding, and the movement-in of going back into oneself - are characteristic not only of the plant or animal organism but of the human being as such. But they are not organic 'processes' we can study like the growth of a plant, nor even movements we are necessarily aware of in any sense at all, for they are themselves basic movements *of* awareness. As such, they may or may not be in accord or harmony with our own 'physiology' in the primordial sense; that is to say, movements which come to rest in a bodying of our being, and which constitute a type of self-originating physiological speech (the *logos* of our *phusis*). This is a bodying, which in the case of the human being implies giving bodily form to what, how and *who* we feel ourselves to *be* at any given time.

Self-psychological dimensions of field-phenomenological medicine

In modern Western culture, the movement of *going in* is associated with a type of introspective or depressive withdrawal which removes us from contact with things and people and leads to the dead end of inner isolation and despair. There is no acknowledgement that the movement in is not only inseparable from the movement of self-unfoldment or 'self-actualisation' that leads us outwards into engagement with the world but its very ground. As in the case of the rooting plant, it is also a going down and going under, movements which also have nothing but negative connotations in our culture. Even as thinking beings distinct from plants, we can no more 'come up' with something without going down into ourselves than a plant can grow upwards and 'come up' with flowers without roots that dig into a fertile soil. In Eastern cultures, the movement in and down found specific forms of *embodiment* in meditational practices and postures which lead to, through and beyond the self. This 'self' however, was at the same time a 'not self' - something fundamentally *other* than the self we ordinarily identify with. It was not, in Buddhist thinking, seen as a singular centre of subjective awareness bounded by the body, but rather as an open-ended or unbounded field of awareness with countless centres, centres which link us, as enlightened beings or Buddhas, with all *other* beings in the indivisible field-continuum of Being that constitutes basic reality. Today, on the other hand, psychoanalytic models of the self have left us with the notion that any *inner* relation we feel to another being, can be nothing more than the psychological internalization of an outer physical relation, the product of a process of 'introjection' or 'projective identification'. From the perspective of field-dynamic phenomenology on the other hand, quite independently of any processes or 'projection' or 'introjection' it is impossible to come face to face with another human being without at the same time coming face to face with ourselves in a new way. The face of the other is always and at the same time another face of the self. The other is not only an 'alter ego', an independent centre of awareness. The other is also an alternate centre of our own larger field of awareness - another self. What we call 'feeling' is not only the expression of a felt resonance with something or someone other than self. It is at the same time an attunement to other selves of our own - an alternative locus of awareness from which we can experience ourselves in a new way and in a new light. Human beings *mean* something to one another not only because of what they do or say to one another but because as beings they already *are* something for one another - they embody other aspects of our own being and attune us to them.

That we ask how someone *feels* with the question 'how *are* you?' or 'how are you *faring*?' (German *Wie geht es dir?* or English *How are you doing?)* points, in Heidegger's understanding to a fundamental 'ontological' unity of being and feeling. "A mood manifests 'how one is' and 'how one is faring'. In this 'how one is', having a mood brings Being to its There." In my view, however, we cannot develop a *feeling* understanding of health and illness without recognizing that at the heart of all human experience is the combination of *familiarity and foreignness* that marks every genuine encounter, not only with others but with ourselves. The sense of foreignness, of *not feeling oneself*, that characterises the experience of *essential dis-ease* can be the starting point, either of disease, or a movement of awareness which leads us to *feeling another self*. Health, from this point of view, is not simply feeling *one-self* again, together with the restoration of a state of bodily 'well-being'. It is a capacity to actively *body* our *inner being* in a way that allows us to assimilate and incorporate new and 'foreign' aspects of ourselves. These are not just other aspects of the self we know but *other selves* - characterised by unfamiliar qualities of awareness latent within our larger identity - that larger field of awareness whose *self-manifestation* we are, and which alone warrants the authentic title of 'self' or 'soul'. We encounter these other selves in other people, which is why we tend to identify them *with* others rather than identifying with them ourselves. Without them however, we would be incapable of 'empathic' attunement to another human being, for this depends on an expansion of our own field of awareness to include those aspects of ourselves that are in *resonance* with the other and constitute our *inner* link to them.

The idea of *one self / one body* has been the ruling self- and body-concept of Western culture for centuries. We speak of "Multiple Personality" only as a *disorder*. Yet we accept without question the body's sophisticated and complex division into multiple organs and cell types. We accept that individuals show different faces, adopt different life roles, or go through subtle changes in personality over time, yet do not see the individual as a family or society of selves but rather as a singular subject or centre of awareness - the conscious ego - with different 'subconscious' layers or 'sub-personalities'. Identity and selfhood in all its diverse aspects, conscious, subconscious and unconscious is seen as the *private property* of a singular ego or "I".

The physical body or *soma* is the 'objective' physically perceived spatial exteriority of the human organism. What we call the psyche is its non-spatial 'subjective' interiority. This non-spatial interiority is no more bounded by the physical body than is the inwardness of the word - its meaning and message - bounded by the physical dimensions of letters on a page. As beings we dwell 'within' our bodies in the same way that we dwell within the word, inhabiting an unbounded, multidimensional world of meaning. The physical body is a living biological language of the human being. But just as a text is the visible two-dimensional surface of a multi-dimensional world of meaning, so is the fleshly text of the human body. The psychic interiority or inwardness of the human organism leads into this world of meaning, one which is limited neither by the boundaries of the physical body *nor* by the outer field of sensory awareness surrounding it. Instead it is an inwardness that both surrounds and permeates this outer field. Understood in this way, the *psyche* is not a physically encapsulated soul but an inwardness *linking us* directly with the inwardness of the things and people we perceive in our external world. The human organism is the instrument or *organon* through which we *translate* our inner relationship to other beings into phenomena manifesting in our outer field of awareness. This inner relationship has the primary character of attunement. We do not first hear someone's words and then deduce from them what they are saying. On the contrary "We hear, not the ear." Our attunement or felt resonance with another human being allows us to hear what they are saying. Our physical hearing then gives form to this attunement as perceived phenomena in our field of sensory awareness - audible words that we hear spoken. We need only remind ourselves, in this connection, of the notorious unwillingness of parliamentarians of all nationalities to listen to what politicians from opposing camps have to say, an unwillingness constantly revealed in their body language through fidgeting, falling asleep, leafing through papers etc. It is not surprising that a German study has revealed that an abnormally large percentage of parliamentary politicians suffer from poor hearing. The *capacity* for attunement that would allow them to hear what others are *saying* rather than 'agreeing' or 'disagreeing' with their propositions and proposals is a capacity that is not merely unexercised but actively inhibited - to such an extent that their organs are functionally affected and their hearing measurably diminished.

Kurt Goldstein was one of the fathers of modern neurology who brought to bear a variety of different holistic, ethical and philosophical perspectives. In his major work entitled "The Organism" he describes how what Heidegger calls 'capacities' are *exercised* in the form of ordered or organised *performances* such as walking or talking, writing or reading, calculating or describing. The latter are in turn a response to a specific environmental field or 'milieu'. If organs are damaged these performances are hindered. Not being able to embody certain capacities through the functioning of its organs the organism cannot 'function' properly ie. cannot respond adequately to a particular *milieu.* This does not mean however, that it is unsuited or unable to respond to the demands of a different milieu. Goldstein's point is that organic 'disease' is not essentially something *intrinsic* to the organism or to the physical body and its organs but rather has to do with the *relationship* between an organism and its milieu. Every change in this relation alters both. For human beings in particular however, loss of ability to exercise their capacities and fulfil their potentials of being through ordered performances in their existing milieu can be experienced as 'catastrophic' threat - tantamount to loss of meaning and loss of being or 'essence'. Echoing the language of Heideggerian ontology Goldstein writes: "This...the organism's being, is its raison d'être. All individual processes take their meaning from and are determined by this being. We describe this as the organism's essence."

"..health is not an objective condition which can be understood by the methods of natural science alone. It is rather a condition related to the mental attitude by which the individual has to value what is essential for his life. "Health" appears thus as a value; its value consists in the individual's capacity to actualise his nature to the degree, that for him at least, is essential. "Being sick" appears as a loss or diminution of value, the value of self-realisation, of existence."

Health in other words, is not the physical or mental ability of an individual to *function* effectively or 'normally' within a pre-given physical or social environment - their milieu. Health is *value fulfillment* - the individual's ability *to find or shape* a milieu *in which* their intrinsic values or potentials of being can be fulfilled as capacities through ordered performances.

Heidegger, Human Genomics
and Health Fascism

According to Goldstein, every organism, including the human organism, dwells in two environments - a 'positive' one which it can respond to effectively through its performances and a 'negative' one which it cannot. Together these make up its milieu. Disease is not the expression of an inborn genetic 'weakness' of the organism in 'adapting' to its environment, but an inability on the part of the individual being to *adapt* that environment to its needs - to find or create the right *milieu* for itself. Stimuli impinging from a negative environment may damage organs, disturb, derange or disable the organism's responses and performances or render them inadequate. The natural response of the individual is to avoid such impingements and/or to alter its positive environment so that it places less demands on functions that are organically impaired - or in danger of becoming so. Neither the bodily and behavioural symptoms of 'disease' necessarily point to organic 'causes', however. Instead they may themselves be healthy and adaptive responses to a negative environment - an attempt to escape that environment or transform it into a life-enhancing milieu. For, the individual too, is on one level a cell within a larger social body that may itself be more or less healthy. The health of the individual and their relation to society cannot therefore be separated from the general health of *human relations* in society

That is why Abraham Maslow rejected "our present easy distinction between sickness and health, at least as far as surface symptoms are concerned. Does sickness mean having symptoms? I maintain now that sickness might consist of not having symptoms when you should."

A sick social organism may reject a healthy cell, treating the individual - or an entire religious, political or ethnic group - as a malignant foreign body or antigen. If the individual suffers or actually becomes sick as a result of this response, is this a healthy response or not? Is it the task of medical science to seek the technological annihilation or 'final solution' to all symptoms of social dis-ease or of an individual's dis-ease with society? Or is its fundamental task to tackle the sicknesses of the social organism itself – those sicknesses *of human relations* that lie at the heart of *both* individual and social ill-health, and one that is no more clearly expressed than in its own sickness-inducing forms of medical diagnosis and treatment?

According to the German-Jewish ethical philosopher Martin Buber, a contemporary of Heidegger, "the sicknesses of the soul are sicknesses of relationship". But what of sicknesses of the body? Is it possible to conceive of an approach to medicine based on relating to the human body as a "Thou" - understanding it as a living embodiment of the individual human being? A form of medicine, in other words, which acknowledged the felt *dis-ease* of the human being, rather than reducing the latter to a medically-labelled and technically treated 'disease'. Or must we, in the name of medical 'science', continue to reduce both the human being and the human body itself to an "It"? Over the last two or three decades it has become hardly possible to even raise fundamental questions of this sort. The media regularly report new discoveries of a gene for this and a gene for that. Whole books are published with titles such as "How the brain thinks" - as if it were human brains or bodily organs rather than human beings that think and feel, see and hear. As humanity begins its journey into the 21st century genetic medicine has become the scientific religion of the new millennium, with the human genome as its god, and the bio-tech labs as its corporate temples. I write on the morning after Clinton and Blair transformed themselves into political worshippers at the feet of this corporate religion and its idols - announcing the successful mapping of the human genome as a technological triumph for mankind and heralding the 'good news' of the benefits it would bring. But the purpose of this essay is not merely to raise questions of 'medical ethics' regarding the *application* of biotechnology, but rather to question its essential truth - the understanding on which it is founded of the human body, the human being, and of the nature of disease itself.

Are we, for example, to understand the human body as a genetic machine in need of repair, or as a living biological language of the human being - its fleshly text? If the latter, then arrogant headlines such as "Decoding the Book of Life" should give us serious pause for thought. For we understand a book by *reading* it i.e. by recognising that the printed page is the two-dimensional surface of a multi-dimensional body of meaning. We do not 'decode' a book by chemical analysis of its ink and paper, by subjecting it to X-rays or by using computers to mathematically 'map' the relationships between the ink marks on the page. A long tradition of Jewish thought holds that the Torah has several quite distinct levels and layers of meaning, not all immediately visible or comprehensible through its surface structure - let alone reducible to it. There are urgent reasons for once again invoking this tradition and its key metaphors - the book as a body of meaning and the body as a fleshly text. For biological medicine, despite its scientific pretensions, is itself based on a quite a different set of metaphors: the body as a biological machine, as a creation of our 'immortal' genes and the instrument for their survival. As for disease, the ruling metaphor of modern medicine would have us believe that this is the work of malignant *foreign bodies* in the form of micro-organisms, cancerous cells or errant genes.

National Socialism, understanding itself as politically applied biology made ample use of this metaphor to 'diagnose' the degenerative disease afflicting the social organism and determine its causes - namely the 'cancerous' and genetically sickly *foreign body* represented by the 'sickly' Jew. National Socialism was based quite explicitly on a *biomedical model* of social disease and its cure. This model was ruthlessly applied, and is still applied today. We know that not only Hitler, but Churchill, Kellogg and others, besides being anti-Semites, were proponents of racial eugenics. We know too, that as late as 1942, leading American medical journals promoted the idea of 'mercy killing' of 'incurable' mental patients. How many of us, however, know that in the 1990's the US government launched a 'violence initiative' aimed at proving the *biological and racial basis of inner-city violence*. And how many of us are aware that 'scientific' medical treatment is itself the fourth largest cause of death in the Western world.

There is a tendency to think of National Socialist ideology as having been an ideological hodgepodge of German romanticism and racist 'pseudo-science'. However, it is also true that the likes of anti-smoking campaigns, the fetishism of 'natural health' and a healthy 'lifestyle' were first bullishly promoted and propagandised in Hitler's Germany. This state-sponsored New-Age style health *faddism*, however, went along with the most sinister form of eugenic health *fascism*, one which finds its contemporary echo in genomics and commercially promoted genetic testing. National Socialist ideologists had appropriated for themselves a powerful cultural counter-movement to *mechanistic* understandings of life and science that had begun in the 1890's and which prepared the ground for serious new 'holistic' approaches to biology - notably those of Uexküll, Driesch and that of the Jewish neurologist Kurt Goldstein. What is less well-known is that it was above all Himmler and the SS who, from 1936 onwards, sought to *purge* German biology of the influence of 'holism' and to replace it with a strictly 'scientific' and 'empirical' approach - in the interests of racial hygiene. Hitler himself compared the "discovery of the Jewish virus" with the work of empirical scientists such as Pasteur or Koch. And according to Peter Breggin, author of *Toxic Psychiatry*, the idea that the lives handicapped or mentally ill were not worth living also influenced the work of the German psychiatrist Ernst Rudin, much respected by Hitler.

The new and insidious form of *health fascism* that we are confronted with today is, of course, untainted by any such associations with Nazi psychiatrists and instead shrouds itself with an aura of medical and scientific respectability. Constant ideological promotion of the myth that mental illness is 'all in the genes' or 'all in the brain' has become an accepted or acceptable proposition, not least the use of psychoactive medications which do not 'correct' the (still-unproven) chemical imbalances supposed to be responsible for 'mental illness' - but create such imbalances by design -

through down-regulating the normal activity of neural receptors for particular neurotransmitters, and in this way thus creating dependency and other effects. Breggin and many others have described the unprecedented and still-growing *epidemic* of drug-induced addiction, dementia and dysphoria created by the prescription or forced use of legal, psychopharmaceutical medications, such as brain-dulling and emotionally anaesthetising 'antipsychotics', highly addictive 'anxiolytic' benzodiazepines (which often cause far more acute symptoms of agitation and anxiety than those for which they were prescribed) and antidepressants - which can not only produce suicidal thoughts but are also thought to be partly responsible for many high-school shooting and other acts of extreme violence. Millions suffer the equivalent of a chemical lobotomy or incarceration in the equivalent of a chemical concentration camp through the use of mind-numbing antipsychotics.

As for the idea that we can use genetic engineering to eugenically 'breed out' predispositions to illnesses such as schizophrenia and to undesirable behaviours such as criminality, and instead 'breed in' desirable qualities such as 'intelligence' is not only intellectually bankrupt and morally suspect but poses, in itself, grave *biological* dangers. Not only does it forget that terms such as 'schizophrenia', 'criminality' or 'intelligence' are not, in the first place, empirical givens, but *socio-linguistic* terms which themselves evolve and change over time and whose meaning is open to interpretation (would coolly calculated military violence for example, be included in the 'violence' that the new eugenicists would seek to breed out, or would their efforts rather be focussed on problematic, poverty-ridden inner-city blacks?). In the second place, it assumes that *seemingly* negative expressions of innate biological predispositions can be eliminated without at the same time eliminating their positive counterparts. The link between genius on the one hand, and melancholia or 'manic depression' on the other has been recognised throughout human history. A world without a *potential* 'idiot' or 'madman' would be a world without a potential creative genius. A world without the emotional openness and *greater-than-average* 'emotional intelligence' of children and adults with Down's syndrome would be a poorer world not a healthier one. So-called 'abnormal' genes in other words, provide a necessary *biological* balance to dominant social concepts of 'normal' behaviour.

The new gene-therapeutic approach to 'curing' disease is motivated by the same desire for economical 'quick-fix' solutions to any disorders or illness which threaten to disrupt the 'normal' economic functioning of human being in the global capitalist system. In other words, the idea of finally eliminating all diseases through manipulating our DNA has as its covert aim the removal of all somatic and behavioural expressions of the stress, dis-stress and *dis-ease* engendered by capitalism itself. Yet even the very belief that manipulation of our genetic code can actually work is absurd. It is equivalent to believing that by eradicating or manipulating our linguistic code - for example certain combinations of letters used in swear words or 'politically incorrect' language - we can remove the anger that people use them to express. The likely result - for which there is already growing evidence - is the development of new and unforeseen iatrogenic diseases.

Medical science prides itself in dealing only with the 'objective' measurable aspects of disease - blood pressure and hormone levels, presence or absence of infection or inflammation etc. But whilst blood pressure can be measured, how are we to measure the patient's accumulated life-pressures? And whilst heart-rate can be measured how are we to measure 'heart-break' or 'loss of heart'? The patient's personal experience of dis-ease, whether in the form of pain or discomfort, emotional distress or physical disability, *is not in itself anything measurable*. Healing too, involves a host of *immeasurable* dimensions - not least the relationship of physician and patient on both a mental, emotional and organismic level. Unfortunately, conventional medical practice is only slowly coming to an appreciation of these immeasurable dimensions of health and healing. Rather than understanding the disease as an expression of the human being, the human being is reduced to a case of the disease. But as was noted in the book "Doctors of Infamy": "There is not much difference whether a human being is looked on as a 'case' or as a number to be tattooed on the arm. These are but two aspects of the faceless approach of an age without mercy... This is the alchemy of the modern age, the transmogrification of subject into object, of man into thing against which the destructive urge may wreak its fury without restraint."

It is not the individual doctor who is at fault, but the fact that medical science still rests on an essentially erroneous understanding of the human body - one which ignores its organic connection to the *human being*. Stripped of this connection, the life of the body itself ceases. It becomes a mere corpse - the original meaning of the Greek word *soma*. It might therefore be better if patients carried labels with the message to physicians: "Warning, human being inside" or "Not just some-body, *my* body".

Widespread sickness remains a major economic threat to a well-functioning global capitalism machine, revealing the spiritual malaise and poverty it generates. But paradoxically, it is also a source of corporate profit for the biotech shareholders and the whole medical-pharmaceutical complex. No wonder then, that genetic medicine, promising as it does not only a new and most lucrative source of corporate healthy industry profit, but - along with the robotisation of the human being under the name of 'transhumanism' - is vaunted as the technological salvation of mankind from all illness. At the same time, the nasty word 'eugenics' has been conveniently erased from the language of genetic medicine, along with any mention of some of its Nazi and U.S. advocates.

What is called the 'Holocaust' marked a historic turning point in which Germans rather than Jews were turned into the ultimately evil 'other'. But the paranoid idea of illness as something un-natural or 'other', caused by alien or malign 'foreign bodies', rather than being an expression of broader life context and conditions does also have a genuine phenomenological basis. When we are ill our bodies and minds do indeed feel 'other' or 'foreign' to us. But the fetish made of the body's immunological 'defences' against malign foreign bodies ignores the empirical fact that our bodies depend for their life on hosts of microorganisms and are regularly exposed to pathogenic viruses and bacteria without any ill effect. Indeed recent studies have shown that today, in contrast to the necessary use of pesticides for epidemic control in German labour camps, it is an exaggerated obsession with hygiene that prevents children developing a natural immunity to such pathogens and has led to the high incidence of such diseases as asthma and childhood diabetes.

Yet there is, I believe, a deeper meaning to the military metaphors of immunology, which springs from our concepts of personal identity. This has to do with the body as body-ego, and the attempt to defend the ego or "I" from new and hitherto foreign dimensions of its own experience and *identity*. The linguistic ego is a subject 'immune' from its verbs and objects. We say "I feel or think X", "I saw or heard Y" as if the identity of the "I" in question remained forever unaffected and unchanged by what it experiences. In dreams on the other hand, *what* we experience goes together with changes in *who* we experience ourselves to be - in our bodily sense of self. In illness too, it is not just what or how we feel that alters but how *we* feel - for we do not 'feel ourselves'.

Both dream symbols and disease symptoms are, I believe, ways of giving symbolic expression to actual or potential changes in our sense of self and our way of relating to others. From this point of view, it makes no more sense to regard disease as an unnatural disruption of health than it does to regard dreaming as an unnatural disruption of sleep. Our current view of illness, however, is as outdated as the scientific view of dreams before Freud - seeing it as an intrinsically meaningless threat to our well-being rather than a natural and meaningful mode of expression of our inner being, reminding us in a bodily way of our own unfelt feeling and unfulfilled potentials of being. The Jungian psychologist Arnold Mindell has written about the connection between illness and what he calls the 'dreaming body', showing through countless case studies how by encouraging patients to feel their symptoms in a more rather than less intense way, to amplify their own pain or distress, the symbolic nature of these symptoms suddenly becomes clear and profound healing changes are precipitated.

The basic motto of Mindell's work is 'feeling not healing'. In contrast, the search for health and healing as an ersatz for feeling has today given rise to a whole range of complementary therapies in addition to those of conventional medicine. This is nothing new. National Socialism was itself essentially an ideology of health which did its utmost to promote both conventional and complementary forms of healing. The idea of a "war" on cancer began with the National Socialists whilst on the other hand, herbal medicines were grown in the field around Dachau to be tried out on concentration camp inmates. The most aggressive anti-smoking campaign in history was launched by the National Socialist government, and "New German Therapy" embraced all the countless naturopathic and "New Age" therapies we see today. All this in support of the health of the German worker and German industrial machine.

The motto 'heal rather than feel' is most appropriate in any society which defines health as *functionality*, using medicine to suppress the body's own expressions of dissent against 'normal' life conditions. The greater the underlying sickness of society and social relationships, the less people feel able to fulfil their own individual values or potentials of being, and the greater the fetish made of health and 'well-being'. Health 'faddism' today does indeed conceal a new and disguised form of health fascism. Genetics has become the secular religion of 'globalisation' because biological medicine and psychiatry offer not only a lucrative source of corporate profit but also a seemingly fail-safe form of social engineering to be achieved by *medicalising and medicating* the social dis-ease and distress generated by the global capitalism. Hence the extraordinary hypocrisy of a society which seeks to protect children from drug dealers whilst officially dealing drugs to them to remove signs of 'abnormal' or 'disruptive' behaviour in schools ie. the ever-growing prescription of anti-depressants and of Ritalin - itself an amphetamine of the same sort dealt on the streets.

All this is of course justified in the name of a 'science' whose most fundamental assumptions are themselves rarely considered, and which both medical ethics and religious thought have proved incapable of challenging in a fundamental way. At the heart of this science is a naively literalistic view of the relation between language and life. From this literalistic perspective, a child with earache who woke up in the morning and said to its mother that an elephant had stepped on its ear would be treated as asserting an empirically and therefore 'scientifically' false proposition. Science identifies truth with the literal truth and 'verifiability' of verbal propositions, not with the metaphorical truth communicated *dia-logos*, through the word rather than in it. In a reductionistic parody of that historic Christian metaphor - the Word become Flesh - the language of the body too is seen only in literalistic terms. The earache *itself,* like all other 'words' of the flesh, is understood merely as a literal fact rather than as a bodily metaphor, as a symptom with identifiable causes that can be cured and without any symbolic meaning transcending those causes. Both the psychotic who claims that there is a bomb in his stomach and the psychiatrist who dismisses this claim take the statement literally rather than metaphorically - both are victims of what Fiumara has called the prevailing *pathology of literalism* that permeates medicine. The child who develops a tummy ache to deal with her fears of going to school may have a *real* tummy ache indeed not just an imagined one, just like the stressed-out manager with a real and not imagined ulcer. But that real tummy ache is not just a biological fact but a living biological metaphor.

Susan Sontag has questioned the idea of 'illness as metaphor', arguing that its danger lies in that it 'blames' the illness on the patient rather than on some biological cause, and can prevent them from seeking 'proper' medical treatment. But the very idea that illness is something blameworthy needs questioning in the first place. Do we blame people for having nightmares or seek to understand the genuine fears and feelings underlying them? Sontag does not question the ruling metaphors of medicine itself, but instead accepts unquestioningly, the literalistic approach to truth in which they are disguised. Paradoxically, it is the culture of scientific literalism that itself *generates* a basic pathological *dis-ease* in human beings - an incapacity to adequately metaphorise and metabolise their own inner life. Fiumara warns that:

"Literal language might even become the almost exclusive means for being with others and sharing life's vicissitudes; it may sadly be the case that whenever a more personal language is used, the environment tends not to respond, as if the individual were non-existent. To adhere to a literalist language is perhaps to try desperately to be normal...In whatever contexts literalness is at a premium there are positive reinforcements for adaptation to a standard vocabulary..."

"...expressions of rage and hatred may even come to constitute rare opportunities for the experience of depth and intimacy; the literalist cultural atmosphere may thus be suddenly shattered with paradoxical 'relief' for the interlocutors engaged in it. To obtain a stronger contact recourse is made to metaphors triggering hostility which in turn can elicit signals of personalised intentions otherwise concealed."

Illness and depression too (not to mention mass deaths through diseases such as AIDS) may increasingly serve as the only vehicles for the metaphorical expression of individual and social dissent - an outer life no longer worth living due to poverty and exploitation or an inner life muted by the pathology of literalism. Is there any answering word to this culture of verbal literalism and the medical literalism of the fleshly word? Religious languages have been the traditional repository of metaphorical meanings expressive of an inner life irreducible to biological givens. But religious fundamentalism, Christian, Jewish and Islamic, with their literalistic understanding of the Bible, Torah and Koran now present merely a counter-cultural mirror-image of the literalism of science itself. Ethical discussions of the relation between biology, evolution and human 'values' present the latter as if they were disembodied cultural or spiritual phenomena bearing no *intrinsic* relation to our biological life. The understanding of human values as shared potentials of being *embodied* in our relationships with other human beings instead gives way to the general mythology that human consciousness and values are mere biological epiphenomena - a mere by-product of the human body and its biology.

It was Heidegger, who, despite his notorious period of involvement with National Socialism, challenged the *racial-biological* elements of National Socialist ideology in a more fundamental way than any other thinker - resulting in his outright denunciation by the chief Nazi 'philosophers'. It was Heidegger who warned prophetically of the coming age of cybernetics and genetic engineering, an age in which calculative, technological thinking would come to dominate both human language and human life to such a ubiquitous extent as to constitute a new and insidious totalitarianism.

Heideggerian thinking *was and remains* the only thinking capable of challenging the 'scientific' foundations of biological materialism race-genetic ideology, genetic medicine - not to mention the increasingly dangerous encroachment of cybernetics and 'Artificial Intelligence' in all areas of human life. And indeed, what could be more 'artificial' than the idea that 'intelligence' can be reduced to a set of calculative algorithms. The transhumanist technological fantasy of creating conscious 'spiritual machines' reflects nothing more than the reduction of the human being to a machine, and the reduction of thinking to pure calculation.

Organismic Therapy
as Medicine beyond Medicine

A truly phenomenological medicine can only be conceived and practiced as a 'meta-medicine' or 'medicine beyond medicine'. Unlike modern and traditional *medicines*, conventional and complementary *medicines*, Western and Eastern *medicines*, what I call meta-medicine questions our basic ethical and philosophical presuppositions concerning the nature and aims of *medicine as such*. Such presuppositions include the belief, for example that 'illness' and 'health' are opposites, that illness is 'bad' and health 'good', that the purpose of medicine is to seek the causes of illness and provide cures, that the 'cause' is a malign foreign body or foreign spirit, and the cure its elimination, excision or exorcism.

The practical focus of meta-medicine is not the supposed 'causes' or 'cures' of disease, but the individual's felt dis-ease and the meaning it holds for them. Meta-medicine is founded on the acknowledgement that there is *meaning* in illness and challenges the medicalisation and medication of dis-ease and distress. It questions the pathologisation of human suffering and disease symptoms, understanding them instead as symbols of a deeper *pathos* (Weizsäcker). It concurs with Illich in understanding suffering itself not as passive victimhood but as *responsible activity* - for it is our capacity to actively bear and body a felt sense of dis-ease that allows suffering to become the healing source of a new sense of wholeness. Meta-medicine adopts for medicine Mindell's motto of 'feeling not healing' - seeing the fundamental task of the physician as one of helping the patient to *feel* their symptoms more not less, and in this way feel more in them - to feel their meaning.

Meta-medicine also transcends the theoretical, practical and institutional separation between psychoanalysis and psychotherapy on the one hand, and somatic medicine on the other, regarding 'psyche' and 'soma', bodyhood and behaviour as twin expressions of the *human organism*. It does not identify the human organism with the physical body as perceived from without but with the body as we experience it from within - with the felt or sensed body.

From this new meta-medical perspective, bodily disease, depression and death itself are not seen as deviations from a healthy state of bodily well-being but as *meaningful* dimensions of a health *process* through which we can become more 'whole' as human beings. The nature of the *illness process* as part of this health process is understood in an ontological way - as a process in which 'not feeling ourselves' is only truly completed when we begin to 'feel another self'.

Healing is no longer identified with mental, emotional or bodily 'recovery' but rather with *self-discovery* - the birth of a *newly felt bodily sense of self*. The *military* metaphors of modern medicine are replaced by the metaphor of *maieusis* - the physician as *midwife*. Illness is understood as a form of gestation in which the patient is pregnant with a new bodily sense of self. Different forms of meta-medical therapy would no longer have the aim of artificially terminating this pregnancy, or interfering with the gestation process. For again, the essential aim of meta-medicine is not *heal* the patient's disease or 'pathology' but help them to *feel* their inner dis-ease. Meta-medicine does not seek to *change* the patient's bodily condition but help the patient *be changed* by it - to discover *more* of themselves through it. Through becoming more authentically whole in this way, efficacious healing in the ordinary medical sense would come about automatically.

In meta-medicine, the patient-physician relationship is intrinsic to the therapeutic process, not an add-on dimension of 'bedside manner' or professional 'listening skills' designed only to give patients the superficial *impression* of being genuinely heard.

"Man can be an individual only in unity with the other...[With patients] this unity will be effective only if it is not a pseudo-unity, a merely external relationship, but if it is a real renewing of lost communion." Goldstein

The practical methods of meta-medical therapy that I have developed are all dependent on the inner relationship of practitioner and patient - the capacity of the practitioner to fully receive and respond to the inner dis-ease of the patient as a human being rather than reducing it to a medically labelled disease of the body or mind. The practitioner's most vital instrument in this process is not their knowledge of or about the body but the wordless knowing of their own organism itself. By allowing their own organism to 'resonate' directly with that of the patient, the practitioner learns to identify organismically with the patient's dis-ease, and to respond to it directly from the healing depths of their own being. Both deep listening and intensive silent eye-contact with the patient play an important role here. When people feel unwell they also 'sound' and 'look' unwell. Their deepest desire is to be fully *heard and seen* as human beings, not treated as 'cases'. They desire that their own suffering be *felt* by another human being - not in order that the other should magically heal and eliminate it, but in order to receive the courage to *feel* it more themselves. To listen to a patient in a therapeutic way is not merely to give them time but to patiently bear with them - helping them bear their suffering and in this way transform it, giving birth to a new inner bearing towards life. "A dispostion can confine man in his corporeality as in a prison. And yet it can also carry him through corporeality as one of the paths leading out of it." Heidegger

Only by learning to actively *bear and body* their felt-disease can the patient's need to express it symbolically through somatic symptoms be removed. In this way - and in this way only - do the bodily or behavioural symptoms that the patient presents with also become unnecessary as a medium of communication, a way to be heard, seen and felt by other human beings. The human body does not 'have' a language - it *is* a living biological language of the human being. This language, like others serves a communicative purpose and therefore healing is also necessarily a communicative *process*. What distorts all human communication, above all that between physician and patient, is the tendency to *react* to others without the restraint necessary to first fully *receive* the other into one's being.

Drugs and gene-therapies are no substitute for communicative healing of this sort - the *communion* that results from the patient being fully received as 'some-body' and not just as a 'talking head' with bodily complaints. If the patient is not received as some-body but merely as 'a body' they are effectively treated 'nobodies', their body and its problems reduced to an *It* - a clinical body-object with which they have nothing to do except submit to the recommended 'treatment'.

That patients should be so 'treated' is a symptom of a social disease, an iatrogenic pathology that mankind has yet to confront - preferring to maintain its addiction to current forms of medical treatment. The greater the impersonal technical sophistication of these treatments, however, the more they function as a form of *institutionalised health engineering* designed to alleviate the more fundamental sickness of human relations in capitalist society. The treatments themselves produce more forms of sickness than those they seek or claim to 'cure'. One need only think of the debilitating or suicide-inducing effects of psychiatric drugs, the 'superbugs' which now infect one out of ten surgical patients in the UK, and the deaths already caused by experiments in gene-therapy: the latest flagship enterprise in *corporate health profiteering*. The new 'health fascism' is already with us, and the hidden holocaust it threatens to inflict has already commenced. It is no accident that people suffering the long-term effects of medical-psychiatric treatments reliant on pharmaceutical drugs call themselves 'survivors'.

When will patients, physicians and politicians alike recognise that the medical-psychiatric crisis afflicting market economies worldwide is nothing that can be resolved by new ways of funding and delivering 'quality' health services, whether public or private. Such topical 'issues' mask the far deeper questions raised by Heidegger in the *Zollikon Seminars*, and heralds a far deeper crisis of belief - a critical turning point in our understanding of the very nature of 'health' and 'illness'. For the critical turn to occur however, requires a fundamentally new understanding of what 'health' and 'illness' essentially *are*, and a new understanding too, of what constitutes 'scientific method' in medicine. The unfulfilled heritage of the *Zollikon Seminars* lie in the seed of thought that Heidegger planted for a *qualitative* revolution in medicine - one not based on new forms of *quantitative* measurement and testing, on impersonal technologies and dehumanising treatments, but on the *quality* of the time that physicians grant to their patients, and the *qualitative depth of awareness* they are trained to bring to their work.

When Freud was 82 years old he formulated what he called the *second fundamental principle of psychoanalysis* - one whose implications have been largely ignored. According to this principle, what is truly *psychical* manifests itself primarily in what were previously considered merely as parallel or 'concomitant' *somatic* phenomena. The 'unconscious' in other words, is nothing essentially biological or psychical but a *somatic psyche*. Meta-medicine understands the physical body (*Körper* or *soma*) as the outwardly perceived form of the human *organism*, with the *psyche* or *soul* being its inwardly felt interiority. The organism *as such* is a *somatic psyche* or *psyche-soma* (Winnicott). It is made up of patterned tonalities of awareness with their own field-patterns and qualities, their own resonances and dissonances, and their own *felt* bodily shape and substantiality. The organism is the musical instrument or *organon* with which we translate feeling tones into cell and muscle tone, their resonant or dissonant patterns into mental and motor patterns.

In contrast to *this* understanding of the psyche and soma as unitary aspects of the human *organism*, talk of the unity of 'body', 'mind' and 'spirit' effectively reduces the organism to a mere assemblage of separate parts. As for the *relation* of soul and body or psyche and soma, it makes no sense to speak of the 'psychogenic' or 'psychosomatic' *causation* of organic disease. For the relation of *psyche* and *soma* as twin aspects of the human organism is not fundamentally a causal relation but a linguistic one. The *psyche*, as the felt *interiority* of the organism, is not same thing as the organic interiority of the body as perceived from without. The latter reveals nothing but a mere *corpus* or *Körper* - the root meaning of *soma*. The psychical interiority of the organism is comparable to the inwardness of the word. The physical body, as its perceived exteriority, is its fleshly text or corpus. The essential relation of psyche and soma is not a causal but hermeneutic and musical one - the relation of a visible text to its felt dimensions of *meaning*, and of a word to its felt inner *resonances*.

As Foucault put it "To ask what is the essence of a disease is like asking what is the nature of the essence of a word." Our felt understanding of the sense or meaning of a word always has to do with connotations that transcend its given meaning or denotation. Just as the same words can have a different felt meaning to different people, so can the same disease symptoms. This felt meaning may not however be manifest, visible, or expressible. It belongs to the realm of unformulated experience. But for what Foucault describes as the clinical gaze what counts is only what is visible - manifest or expressible.

In Diagram 1 below, the black squares represent manifest or expressible symptoms in the way these are perceived by the physician - as diagnostic signs of a generic disease type. The figures within the squares however, represent the varying 'shapes' of different patients' felt experience of the same symptoms or disease. The shaded area within these figures represents their felt dis-ease as such - the organismic field-state that finds expression in their symptoms.

Diagram 1

patient 1   patient 2

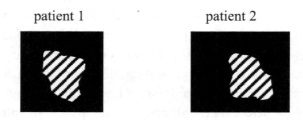

Diagram 2 represents the way in which a patient's felt dis-ease can take on the form of a typical disease pattern. This may happen either because the disease pattern is identified by the physician as a possible cause of their symptoms or because the patient has already begun to medically interpret their felt dis-ease as a sign of some incipient disease - knowing that only in this way will it receive recognition by the physician.

Diagram 2

Conventional medicine, not only orthodox medicine but also many forms of alternative medicine, sees symptoms as literal signs of an underlying somatic or psychological pathology rather than as metaphorical signifiers of a felt sense of dis-ease. The physician's first act is to separate the patient as a human being from their symptoms, to objectify the latter and to reduce them to signs of some 'thing' lying behind them. Diagram 3 is a model of the traditional "We-It" relationship between physician and patient, in which the physician's principle is to separate the patient's felt dis-ease from their manifest medically-recognized disease symptoms and turn the latter into an "It" - some 'thing' that is 'wrong' with the patient and that can be turned into an object of clinical diagnosis and treatment.

Diagram 3

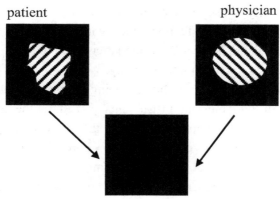

patient physician

manifest symptoms

Meta-medicine marks a break with all forms of diagnosis that are not based on a direct *organismic resonance* with the patient's felt body and the felt dis-ease it expresses. Organismic resonance is not the same thing as emotional empathy. A physician or psychologist can register a sign of somatic discomfort or emotional distress in a person, and feel empathy or compassion for them, without in any way resonating with its unique tonality: the 'felt quality' or 'field-quality' of *this* patient's discomfort or distress, *this* person's pain or despair, this person's *felt body* and this person's *felt dis-ease*.

The practice of meta-medicine is *organismic therapy* - based on the therapist's capacity to use their own organism to sense and *resonate with* the felt body and felt dis-ease of the patient.

The *practitioner* of this organismic therapy is someone who can not only bring their felt body into *resonance* with that of the patient but also freely tune, tone and 'play' their own organism as a musical instrument or *organon*. This means using it to emanate feeling tones that not only echo and amplify those of the patient, but also modulate the patient's organismic feeling tones with new and different tones which are *harmonics* of the latter – and thus help bring the patient's organism into harmony.

"The nerves of the two human beings can be compared to chords of two musical instruments placed in the greatest possible harmony and union. When the chord is played on one instrument, a corresponding chord is created by resonance in the other instrument." Tardy de Montravel

Diagram 4 represents a state of organismic resonance between patient and therapist, through which the therapist has achieved a state of *organismic resonance* - gained an inner bodily sense of the patient's felt dis-ease.

Diagram 4

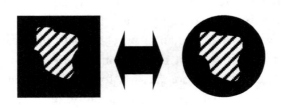

patient   therapist

The principal instrument of meta-medical therapy is the therapist's own organismic awareness. The therapist is one who has transformed their own organism into a new organ of *feeling cognition*, one through which they can sense the unique field-qualities of another person's organism. The medium of this qualitative perception is 'feeling tone'. For like audible voice tones, organismic feeling tones have their own sensual qualities of warmth and coolness, lightness and darkness, just as they also possess different 'elemental' qualities such as fluidity and solidity, airiness or fieriness, different tone 'colours', expressed in and through different sound 'shapes', 'timbres' and 'textures'.

A visibly stocky and muscular patient feels light or weightless to the therapist. Though she has a 'sunny' disposition, which can be sensed organismically as radiation of light and warmth it is as if her awareness were constantly streaming outwards towards the world and other people rather than inwards towards her own self. This was reflected in the fact that though she talked a lot about others and showed great emotional perceptiveness she never spoke directly about her own feelings or her experience of herself. A felt sense develops in the therapist of a hollow quality of the patient's bodily self-awareness - her awareness entirely dwelling on the mental outer surface of her organism and in the outer world, and lacking any centre in its bodily, psychic interiority. Her sparkling eyes and talkative vitality betrayed a lacking field-depth and field-intensity in the patient's inner bodily self-awareness. Her entire awareness of herself seemed outwardly oriented, merged with her awareness of others and head centred rather than inwardly or body centred.

The therapist's direct organismic awareness of the patient was given significance by both her somatic complaints and the verbal information she communicated. In a brief telephone call with this client the therapist got an intuitive sense that the patient was not just alone in the house, but in a sort of vacuum. Later the patient reported that she was indeed alone in the house at the time, but also had, for a change, no external problems, her own or others, to focus her awareness on. It was at this time she experienced a somatic crisis. This took the form of an allergic shock reaction in which her body tissues swelled, she felt like a balloon and due to constriction of her throat it became almost impossible for her to breathe or speak.

The therapist's organismic sense of this crisis was that the patient's body was expanding to fill an external vacuum created by the patient's lack of inner bodily self-awareness. That it was intensifying her bodily self-awareness and using her physical body to substitute for the otherwise non-existent boundary between self and other in her organism or body of awareness. An untrammelled and unmeasured flow of awareness between self and world was physically disrupted through her body making it almost impossible for breath to flow in and out. The shock reaction in other words, was not a response to a specific allergen but her immune system going into hyperdrive in order to compensate for a lack of boundedness in her organism and a lack of differentiation between self and other reflected in her language and way of speaking.

According to Martin Heidegger "We cannot say that the organ has capacities but must say that the capacity has organs...capability, articulating itself into capacities creating organs characterizes the organism as such." Respiration, digestion and metabolism for example, are not merely organic functions of the physical body or *soma* but the *embodiment* of a fundamental *capacity* of our being. These capacities are bodied through the human organism - which, as a *body of awareness*, is the *body* with which the human beings inhale and exhale, digest and metabolise their own *experience* of the world and other beings, drawing from it the raw material with which they reconstitute and transform their *self-experience*. Meta-medicine identifies eight basic dynamics governing the relation between, on the one hand, *organismic capacities* such as inner psychical respiration, circulation and metabolism, and, on the other hand the bodily mental *functions* (including brain functions) that are their outer counterparts.

1. A weakened organismic capacity weakens a bodily function.
2. A weakened bodily function weakens an organismic capacity.
3. A strengthened organismic capacity strengthens a bodily function.
4. A strengthened bodily function strengthens an organismic capacity.
5. A bodily function compensates for an under-active organismic capacity.
6. An over-active bodily function weakens an organismic capacity.
7. A weakened organismic capacity strengthens bodily function
8. A weakened bodily function strengthens an organismic capacity.

This case was a clear example of an organic function (the auto-immune system) compensating for a weak or non-existent psychical capacity to form a firm organismic boundary or skin of awareness of self and of other. Her most continuous somatic symptom was itchy skin eruptions from which she scratched to the point of drawing blood - as if to break into herself from the outside. Biographical questioning revealed that in her childhood the patient had suffered from constant fears of her mother dying while she was at school, confirming the therapist's organismic sense of an absent differentiation of self and a significant other in the form of the mother. This too was related to the deathly hollowness of her organism, which as a vital and formative inner body is also a 'mother-body'. Because of this hollowness, fiery intensities of awareness have not only no firm boundary to contain them but no organismic surface to rise to in the first place. The patient's somatic sensation of intense bodily heat and going 'red in the face' during the somatic crisis allowed her inner fire to condense and rise to a surface rather than being dissipated in the ordinary way as the warmth and light of her normal radiant or sunny disposition. A dream shared by the patient revealed an intense fear of darkness. Her predominant skin symptoms - hot and itchy eruptions - were reminiscent of sunspots - concentrations of heat that made her physically aware of an organismic skin she lacked psychically and made up for through a continuous mental skein of thoughts about others.

Therapy did not take the form of physical diagnosis and treatment, psychological explanations of symptoms or psychoanalytic interpretations focusing on emotional issues and their source in parent-child relationships. The fundamental therapy was the fundamental dia-gnosis - the therapist's capacity to stay with his own felt, organismic sense of the patient's inner vacuum and lack of boundedness - despite all her surface vitality and talkativeness. This in turn induced a state of field-resonance with the patient's own organism – allowing her to feel its hollowness for the first time. The therapist then used his own organism to directly induce a sense of inner warmth in the organism of the patient, helping her to feel her own body not as a vacuum emptied of awareness but as a vessel or hearth - filled with a warm glow of awareness stemming from her own life-fire.

Just as there are organismic counterparts to every organ and physiological function (in this case the skin and auto-immune function) so there are also inner psychical counterparts to physical phenomena such as space and time, closeness and distance, warmth and coolness, light and darkness, lightness and heaviness, sound and density, charge and polarity, electricity and magnetism. This applies also to the elements such as fluidity (water), solidity (earth) and gaseousness (air). The organism is composed of different combinations of these inner energies and elements - qualities of inner warmth and inner light for example. But it is of the utmost importance not to confuse our felt sense of these qualities with bodily sensations of some physical or vital 'energy'. The warmth we feel radiating from a human being for example, is neither a measurable property of their physical body (temperature) nor some mysterious inner energy that we happen to be aware of. It is a quality of their awareness of themselves and the world that others then feel bathed in and warmed by. Just as we can feel inwardly close to someone even though they are miles away, so can our feelings towards someone have a warm quality even though our bodies are freezing. Just as our organism, as a body of awareness, is not less but more fundamentally real than any physical phenomena we are aware of, so are inner closeness or distance, warmth or coolness, lightness and darkness, fluidity or solidity etc. more fundamentally real than their physical counterparts.

When we feel a person's warmth or see the radiance of their gaze we are not speaking of any physical heat or light emanated by their bodies. Nor are we merely speaking metaphorically. To believe so is to imply that the warmth or light we feel emanating from a human being is somehow less real than a measurable temperature of the human body or the measurable light reflected by their eyes. To talk, as many 'New Age' alternative practitioners do, of a person's bodily 'energy' and of 'energy medicine' seems to imbue our felt, organismic sense of other human beings with a more tangible 'objective' reality than a mere 'subjective' feeling about them. At the same time however, it is an evasion of the basic question of what is more real or fundamental - the human body or the human being, energetic relationships between bodies in space and time, or inner relationships between beings. To say that it is 'energy' that links or relates things and people is one thing. Put the other way round, we can say that the essence of energy is *relationality* as such.

The human organism is not an 'energy body' but the instrument through which we embody our *felt relation* to the world and other people. The practice of meta-medicine, as organismic therapy, is effective to the extent that the therapeutic relationship becomes a medium of direct organismic resonance and response to the felt dis-ease of the patient - and to the disturbance this reflects in the patient's own felt relation to the world.

The Principles
of the Field-Phenomenological Method

Phenomenological science is science understood *as* phenomenology. The methodological principles of phenomenological science and research, the so-called 'phenomenological method', must therefore be understood as the essence of scientific method *per se*, not as an alternative to it.

1. The Phenomenological Reduction

Husserl placed the 'phenomenological reduction' at the heart of the phenomenological method, meaning by this the suspension or 'bracketing' of any naturalistic or 'positivistic' mindset which 'naturally assumed' or theoretically posited an objective world of pre-given entities independent of or inaccessible to subjectivity or awareness.

2. The Phenomenological Rule

By the 'phenomenological rule' I refer to Heidegger's principle that "All explanation reaches only so far as the explication of that which is to be explained." The rule demands that before attempting an explanation of a phenomenon we should also bracket pre-conceived ideas of what the phenomenon in question is, and what the term by its designation essentially names. For example, to explain the 'causes' of phenomena such as anxiety, stress or depression and find a 'cure' is to break this rule. For it is to assume, without further ado that we already all know what it is that is designated with the terms 'anxiety', 'stress' and 'depression'. Physical-scientific methods determine in advance which phenomena are deemed scientifically significant and how those phenomena are understood. Thus 'depression' is understood today as a chemical imbalance of the brain even though there have been no experiments done to prove this claim, and no evidence of this 'fact' exists. Despite this, psychopharmacology has gone on to posit explanatory 'causes' of this chemical imbalance and to 'cure' it with drugs. Freud explained the causes of 'hysteria' and claimed to find a cure for it in psychoanalysis. At the time it was taken as a pre-given thing in defiance of the phenomenological reduction. Now the word 'hysteria' no longer even figures in the medical-scientific lexicon, and its existence as a medical disease entity - a 'thing in itself' is doubted. Were the phenomenological rule to have been applied in the first place, the question would not have been 'how to explain the causes of hysteria and cure' it but 'what is hysteria?' i.e. what essentially is the phenomenon that is designated by the word 'hysteria'? This is not the sort of question that can be answered by simply grouping a set of psychiatric symptoms under a common diagnostic term. The question requires us to not only look at the designated phenomenon as a phenomenon - to see what modes of being in the world it brings to light (*phainesthai*). It also requires us to examine the word itself as a word, to be aware not only of its current usage and denotation but of its history and connotations.

3. Phenomenological Reading

If words such as 'depression' or 'hysteria' are taken literally, seen as designations for some underlying disorder or disease, which is taken as a thing in itself, then a patient's symptoms are taken simply as 'signs' of this pre-given thing - the disease or disorder. No attempt is made to read these signs in any other way, to understand their *felt* sense or significance for the patient themselves. Medicine treats symptoms as bodily words without any communicative sense or meaning. It is as if we would seek to understand the meaning or significance of the written or spoken word itself without any regard for what an individual was saying with them. Instead we set about 'scientifically' analysing the physical components of LCD screens, the chemical make up of ink and paper, or the vibrations of sound waves in the air, seeking chemical or vibrational causes for any unusual, 'unhealthy' or 'unsound' language. Reading phenomena, like reading words, is something quite different from turning them into objects of scientific scrutiny or analysis.

4. Phenomenological Relation

The felt sense or significance of a word or phenomenon will vary from person to person, culture to culture. Similarly, our reading of a word or phenomenon is determined by our own relation to it. This does not render all phenomenological insight into something personally or culturally 'relative'. On the contrary, it allows us to become aware of our existing *relation* to specific phenomena, and by altering or deepening that relation to understand them in new and deeper ways. It was Heidegger who first marked out the Phenomenological Relation as a basic principle of the phenomenological method, indicating that the modern terms 'relativity' or 'relativism' conceal the deeper truth that all knowledge is relational. "Knowing is a relation in which we ourselves are related, and in which this relation vibrates through our basic comportment". Reading phenomena like reading words or reading people is impossible without awareness of our own relation to them and without a preparedness to alter and deepen that relation. The principle of the Phenomenological Relation can be summed up as follows: scientific knowledge of relationships *between* phenomena, for example between things and between people, can only be deepened by deepening our own aware relation to them.

It may be objected that the above-stated principles of phenomenological science and the phenomenological method, whilst perhaps suitable for 'qualitative' research in human sciences such as psychology, sociology or anthropology, is nevertheless quite inadequate in dealing with the 'objects' of physical-scientific research – such as light, heat, gravity, time and space etc. To contrast modern scientific methods deriving from the physical sciences with phenomenological science and phenomenological methods is therefore inappropriate - notwithstanding the fact that the human sciences have themselves come more and more under the domination of quantitative methods deriving from the physical sciences. To this objection it is necessary to state a number of further, hitherto unthought and unstated principles of the phenomenological method, undeveloped by Husserl but decisively hinted at by Heidegger. It is only on the basis of these principles that the phenomenological method can be understood as a method fundamental to all the sciences and accomplish its transformation into what I call Fundamental Science.

5. Phenomenological Realism

We see that an object, a tree or table for example, is there. We take this as evidence of its existence. But the existence, 'is-ness' or 'being-ness' of the tree or table that is there – in other words its 'Dasein', 'being there', is not in itself any natural or manufactured 'thing', nor is it the object of any possible visual perception. The German word 'Da' can mean either 'here' or 'there'. As far as we are concerned, we stand here and the object that we see stands there. But our *seeing* of the table is neither here nor there. It is not itself an object we can localize in space, either in the space around us or in some body-object such as eyes, optic nerves or brain. We do not see the object only because it stands in the light. A blind person can be aware of the table or tree, know its shape and sense its distance and in this sense 'see' it, even without functioning eyes. Whether we direct our vision or our thoughts towards the tree or table, turning it into what Husserl called an "intentional object" of consciousness, is irrelevant. For not only our perception of a thing but the very thoughts we have about it arise within a non-localized *field* of awareness. This field of awareness is not itself a possible object of *consciousness* for a 'subject'. It is not in itself an "intentional object". On the contrary, awareness, in its non-local or field character, is the very condition of emergence of any localized objects for any localized subject or 'intentional' consciousness, and thus more fundamentally real than the latter.

6. Phenomenological Reversal

Heidegger designated the non-local or field character of awareness through a poetic use of the words *Feldung* and *Lichtung* - a cleared field or forest 'clearing' in which things stand out in the light and first come to light. Light, as we know, plays a major role in modern physics. Not only Einstein's famous equation but also quantum physics makes it into a linchpin phenomenon for the physical-scientific research of the intimate relationship between matter and energy. But can light be truly regarded as a purely physical phenomenon at all? Things become visible only in the light of our own awareness of them, not simply because they radiate or reflect physical light. Both the *physics* of light and the *neurophysiology* of visual perception still fail to address, let alone answer, the fundamental questions of *optics* - namely, what sort of 'light' is it with which the brain supposedly produces illuminated perceptual *images* of physical objects - not only in the waking state, but also in our dreams? Recent research has shown that a two-way relation exists between brain and eye, the brain actually sending signals via the optic nerve to the eye in waking life as it does when we dream. But even such research offers no answer to the fundamental question, which can be put as follows: what is the relation between our *awareness of light* on the one hand, and the *light of awareness* on the other?

Within the spiritual traditions of the past, light, and with it, enlightenment and illumination, played as central a role as it does in physical science today. Today however, terms such as enlightenment or 'light of awareness' are seen as mere poetic metaphors. In this stance, modern science stands in gross contradiction to itself. More specifically the physics of light stands in gross contradiction to neurophysiology, which claims that what appear as illuminated objects, are images or effigies created by the brain. Classical optics claimed that to explain visual perception, it was necessary to distinguish two types of light - the natural light received by the eye (*lumen*) and the subjective light radiated by the eye (*lux*). The neurophysiological understanding of optical perception is a concealed version of classical optics, recognizing that what we perceive as objects in the world are subjectively projected and illuminated. The cosmologist however, though making use of optical instruments to perceive the stars, decisively ignores all fundamental questions to do with the nature of visual perception as a subjective spatial projection of images, and a subjective projection of spatial distance and depth. Optics, as a science that must seek to unite both

112

'objective' and 'subjective' dimensions of perception, remains the Achilles heel of a purely objectivistic approach to science, requiring from both the physicist and the brain scientist what Heidegger called a type of "double or triple accounting" with regard to the subjective dimension.

"When it is claimed that brain research is a scientific foundation for our understanding of human beings, the claim implies that the true and real relationship of one human being to another is an interaction of brain processes, and that in brain research itself, nothing else is happening but that one brain is in some way 'informing' another. Then, for example, the statue of a god in the Akropolis museum, viewed during the term break, that is to say outside the research work, is in reality and truth nothing but the meeting of a brain process in the observer with the product of a brain process, the statue exhibited. Reassuring us, during the holidays, that this is not what is really implied, means living with a certain double or triple accounting that clearly doesn't rest easily with the much faulted rigor of science."

As Ronchi rightly suggests, ancient physics was closer "in our modern terminology, to the physiology of the senses". Or rather the essential focus of ancient physics was neither human physiology nor the physics of the cosmos *per se*, but man's sentient awareness of the cosmos. Where modern physics speaks of 'light', 'heat', 'gravity' and 'sound' as entities independent of the senses, the focus of ancient physics was on our sentient awareness of light and darkness, warmth and coldness, weight and lightness, as well as of elemental qualities of fluidity or solidity, airiness or fieriness. Dreams made it self-evident to the ancients that sentience in all its forms had an intrinsically subjective character. The change to the modern scientific world view began with optics, which began as a science of visual perception involving an aware and sentient perceiver and has ended up as a wave optics bearing no relation to our own sentient awareness of light (*lumen*) and denying the very existence of a subjective light of awareness (*lux*).

What I call the Phenomenological Reversal is the insight that the term *light of awareness* is no mere metaphor but points to something more real and fundamental than the body's sensory awareness of physical light, even though both physicist and physiologist alike still cling, contradictorily, to the myth that the latter is somehow primary. Behind this insight lies the recognition that awareness as such is not something neutral, a mere passive receptacle of thoughts and perceptions, but something that is always qualitatively coloured, toned and weighted in a particular way.

The *chiasm* fundamental to the Phenomenological Reversal reads:

awareness of light / light of awareness

It can also read:

awareness of forms / forms of awareness,
awareness of weight / weightedness of awareness,
awareness of space / spatiality of awareness,
awareness of time / temporality of awareness.

In each case the Phenomenological Reversal understands the second term in the chiasm as primary rather than secondary. Treating it as a secondary or 'metaphorical' result, as in the case of light, is a logical self-contradiction. It also offends our everyday experience that awareness is always mooded - toned and tuned, coloured and shaped in a particular way. A common sense which knows too that no physical-scientific understanding of light and no neuro-physiological understandings of the brain will ever be able to explain even the simplest phenomena of everyday and 'everynight' consciousness – to say how 'wavelengths' of light become conscious perceptions of colour for example, or how brain activity 'produces' a consciousness of luminous dream landscapes and visions.

The word 'physics' derives from the Greek *phuein* - to emerge or arise. The word phenomenon derives from the Greek *phainesthai* - to come to light. Physical phenomena arise or emerge (*phuein*) as phenomena only within fields of awareness. Doing so, they bring to light (*phainesthai*) specific field-qualities and field-patterns of awareness. It is in the experience of *dreaming* however, that we can actually experience 'physics' as *phusis* or emergence in this sense, experiencing perceived phenomena as a 'coming to light' of particular moods or colourations, forms and figurations of awareness. Only in dreaming have we the opportunity to experience, for example the transformation of a particular bright or dark mood or colouration of awareness into what emerges and appears to us, phenomenally, as the physical image of a bright or dark dream sky or landscape.

Neither Husserl nor Heidegger fully recognized the fundamental scientific implications of the Phenomenological Reversal, for it amounts to a reversal in the understanding of phenomenology itself. With the Phenomenological Reversal goes the understanding that the true focus on phenomenological science, indeed the fundamental nature of reality itself does not consist of physical phenomena such as waves and particles, light and colour, vibration and sound, intensities and polarity, fluid currents and stable forms or patterned structures etc. Rather its focus, and the fundamental nature of reality, is composed of wave and particle-like qualities of awareness, luminosities and colourations of awareness, vibrational pitches and tonalities of awareness, fluid currents and patterned structures of awareness. Fundamental reality does not consist essentially of any sensory physical phenomena we are aware of - but sensual field-qualities and field-patterns *of* awareness. It is this reversal in our understanding of the fundamental nature of reality and of phenomenology itself that accomplishes the transformation of phenomenological science into a Fundamental Science of equal relevance to the human and natural sciences.

7. Phenomenological Reciprocity

Just as Husserl understood consciousness as intentional - consciousness of something, so Freud compared consciousness to a searchlight, something that can be aimed at an object. Physics too, understands light as something that 'travels' in one direction, like the light emanating from a torch or lighthouse beacon. How is it however, with the light of awareness? We do not simply experience the world in the light of our own awareness of it. We also experience ourselves in the light of the things and people around us. As long as we think of awareness as some sort of uni-directional light radiated by a localized source - a conscious subject - we ignore not only its field character but its intrinsically *reciprocal* nature. For wherever, whatever and whoever we direct the 'searchlight' of our consciousness towards, at another level we are constantly *aware* of ourselves in the light of all that we behold around us. Whether it is a thing or thought, a place or person, a fact or feeling, a past or future event that we direct our attention to, makes no difference. Our awareness of ourselves is altered in the light of whatever it is we are aware of. Not only can we not witness an accident or crime without feeling changed, if only thankful not to have been involved, we cannot so much as walk down a street or stand next to another person without our self-awareness being subtly altered by them. Standing next to a short person we feel taller. Walking down a shabby street in smart clothes, we may feel out of place. Our awareness of ourselves and of the world are inseparable and in constant reciprocal interaction. Our relationship to both objects and people hinges on the reciprocal character of awareness. What Freud called the 'unconscious' is this other side to his uni-directional searchlight of 'consciousness' - our awareness of ourselves in the light of the things around, or in the light of other people's consciousness of us.

Dreams let in the 'unconscious' because in them the separation between our self-awareness and our awareness of the world, the light of our own consciousness of others, and the light of their consciousness of us, breaks down. In this sense dreaming is indeed a return of the repressed, a return of a repressed reciprocity in which our everyday self-awareness is altered not only in the light of others but in the light of those other parts of ourselves that link us to them within a larger field of 'intersubjectivity'. But the term 'intersubjectivity' is far from adequate for grasping the nature of this field. For it suggests that the reciprocity of awareness is the product of an interaction between two pre-given subjects, each with their own distinct consciousness of self. In fact, that very consciousness of self is itself a product of an ongoing reciprocity of awareness. It is the 'particle' dimension of awareness, whose complementary *wave* character allows a two-way flow, allowing our awareness to merge with that of others and form ever-changing *field patterns* of identity that are the *private property* of neither one self or subject nor the other. The 'light of awareness' is no metaphor. It is relativity theory and the quantum physics of light that are the metaphors - scientific metaphors of a complex and multi-dimensional *field-dynamics* of awareness as such.

8. Phenomenological Retrieval

Our normal view of consciousness is that it is simply a receptacle for our sensory perception of physical objects and their qualities. In Freud, however, we find an unusually contrasting definition of consciousness as "a sense organ for the perception of psychical qualities". By "psychical qualities" Freud is thinking in particular of the emotions and of experiences of pain and pleasure. Fundamental Science extends the concept of psychical qualities to include all the *psychical counterparts* of *physical* qualities such as light and darkness, warmth and coldness, distance and closeness. How close or distant we feel from another person, the lightness or darkness of their mood, and the warmth or coolness of our relation to them, are, in our everyday experience, not less but *more* fundamentally real to the human being than measurable distance in space that separates us from them, the intensity of the ambient light they reflect, or the measurable temperature of the human body. Nevertheless, these physical parameters are meaningful to us as expression of their psychical counterparts. If we are separated by a physical distance from someone close to us, we may feel either less close or, conversely, even closer to them psychically than before. The meaning or sense that physical qualities and relationships have for us, has to do with how they reflect or refract their psychical qualities. The latter are not merely subjective qualities induced by *sensory* experiences - we do not feel warm towards another person just because we sense warmth in our own bodies or in theirs. On the contrary, our bodies may measurably warm up as a result of feeling warmed by the presence of another human being. To speak of 'psychical' as opposed to 'physical qualities' should not be taken to imply some form of psycho-physical dualism. For one thing physical qualities are themselves qualities of our own sensory awareness, and in this sense also 'psychical'. Nevertheless, any *sensory qualities we are aware of* through our bodies remain distinct in character from those *sensual qualities of awareness* which determine our relation to other *beings* - the warmth with which we regard them or the closeness we feel to them for example.

Perhaps the single most important misconception of phenomenology is that its focus lies on our direct *sensory* experience of the world rather than on the felt meaning or *sense* of that experience. The Phenomenological Reversal allows us to fully overcome this misconception, and to appreciate instead that lived experience, and the felt sense or meaning of that experience are quite distinct. Meaning or sense has to do with the psychical qualities that find expression as phenomena in lived sensory experiences. All physical phenomena we are aware of serve as *signifiers* of psychical qualities - that is to say, of qualitative dimensions *of* awareness. The latter constitute the felt meaning or *sense* of physical events and experiences.

What we call 'life' is essentially an ongoing process of 'semiosis' - which I understand not just as a process of 'sign making' but as the overall process by which we *make sense* of our lived experience. We do so in two primary ways. One way is to signify felt senses (for example signifying the sense of warmth we feel towards another person through our words, deeds or body language). Another way is by feeling sense or significances (for example, sensing in another person's words, deeds or body language a feeling of warmth towards us). What I call the Phenomenological Retrieval is the process by which, in *recollecting* our lived experiences, we retrieve a felt sense of its significance, which we might not have had at the time. A manager coming home from a hard day's work at the office for example, may be aware of sensations of tension in the neck or pain in their head, and say that they have a headache. The headache is then constituted mentally as objectified physical and bodily phenomenon - a thing in itself. Alternatively, the same manager might come home from the office, aware of the same bodily sensations of tension and pain, and in *recollecting* all that took place in the office that day, *retrieve a felt sense* of a tense mood or mode of awareness that permeated the atmosphere in the office that day, one that was mentally ignored as people got on with their tasks, but which found expression in people tensing themselves up in bodily ways, feeling emotionally 'stressed' and *signifying* their own tension and stress by behaving in particular ways. Continuing to recollect the day's events, and to dwell within their felt sense of the office atmosphere as an intersubjective 'field-state' of awareness, the manager might then begin to discern some underlying meaning within it - not merely blaming it on the behaviour of those who might be considered its 'cause', but seeing the atmosphere and this behaviour as the indirect expression or 'signifier' of certain unspoken conflicts of interest that were not directly communicated. In doing so, our manager may also come to understand their own role in ignoring these felt resentments and not dealing with the unspoken conflicts, and come to understand their own headache symptoms as a lingering bodily *signifier* of something that had gone amiss - of the still *unsensed significance* of their lived experience of that day and its still unthought or *unsignified sense*.

I use this example to emphasize that Phenomenological Retrieval, like the other principles of the Phenomenological Method, is not merely part of some artificially constructed theory or technique to be applied to academic, philosophical and scientific research. It is itself inherent to and a part of everyday life. In the case of the Phenomenological Retrieval however, it is a part of the process of *making sense* of our lives which people rarely grant *time* for. Instead they leave it to the psychical life of their dreams or the somatic life of their bodies to express the unsensed significance and unsignified sense of their lived experience. But what applies in life, applies also to science. And in both life and science *another* method tends to be applied to make sense of experienced events and phenomena. This other method seeks to fit all experiences into a pre-conceived pattern of signification in which what Gendlin calls felt sense or directly cognized meaning has no role. In the case of the example, a person's behaviour that day is immediately identified as part of their particular pattern of behaviour and taken as further *evidence* of the existence of this pattern. No-one asks what the pattern itself signifies, what it itself might be an expression of. Similarly, if the manager begins to suffer regular and periodic headaches, and because of this goes to see a physician, the latter may take the symptoms as a signifier of some 'thing' - an organic disorder for example - seeking to fit it into some already established pattern of diagnostic signification. The question of what, assuming it exists, the organic disorder might itself be a symbol or signifier of, is not asked.

The assumption is that a phenomenon, taken as a sign, must be a sign of some actual thing or already understood pattern - whether a disease pattern, a market pattern or a pattern of behaviour. In the case of the manager's headaches, the true *sense* of the symptoms as signs does not lie in anything actual but in something still potential - the manager's still undeveloped capacity to consciously retrieve their own felt understanding of their own lived experience and of the 'behaviour patterns' of other employees - and thereby respond to them differently.

9. Phenomenological Re-embodiment

The link between life and scientific research lies in the fact that both are sense-making or semiotic processes. *Semiosis* or sense-making not only shapes our perception of the physical universe but constitutes its fundamental dynamic. The interaction of particles, for example, itself makes *inter-objective* sense of energetic relationships between bodies - bringing them to light as measurable scientific phenomena. It does so in exactly the same way that social events make *inter-objective* sense of *intersubjective* relationships between beings - bringing them to manifestation as observable patterns of human behaviour and interaction. Phenomenological research in the social sciences focuses on the methods of sense-making through which individuals shape their interactions and co-constitute an agreed consensual reality. Phenomenological research in the natural sciences focuses on the sensed psychical counterparts of physical phenomena such as light and colour, sound and resonance, weight and gravity, density and form etc. The exploration is not experimental but meditational, exploring the nature and relationship of these phenomena in the most direct way possible - through the *felt body* of the researcher. As a physical body the human being is a part of nature and intimately connected to the universe as a whole. Only through the field-awareness that belongs to the felt body can

Phenomenological Research explore all those underlying field-dimensions, field-qualities and field-patterns of awareness that find expression in our sensory awareness of the physical universe. The felt body is the *bearer* of those unsensed dimensions of significance and unsignified dimensions of meaning or sense that underlie our experience of both human nature and the natural world. The principle of 'Phenomenological Re-embodiment' affirms the centrality of the felt body of the researcher to the Phenomenological Method and Phenomenological Research. The purpose of the latter is neither to provide a 'descriptive' account of our 'lived experience' nor to enframe it within established patterns of signification but to obtain meditative insights into those unsensed dimensions of significance to which we have access only through *felt sense* and the *felt body*. These are insights no less amenable to mutual validation on the part of independent researchers than those sought through the method of the physical sciences.

Bibliography

Fiumara, G. C. *The Metaphoric Process* Routledge 1995
Garfinkel, Harold *Studies in Ethnomethodology* Prentice-Hall 1967
Gendlin, Eugene *Experiencing and the Creation of Meaning* Northwestern University Press 1997
Goldstein, Kurt *The Organism* Zone Books 1995
Harrington, Anne *Holism in Germany from Wilhelm II to Hitler* Princeton 1996
Heidegger, Martin *Zollikoner Seminare* Klostermann 1994
Heidegger, Martin *The Fundamental Concepts of Metaphysics* Indiana 1995
Heidegger, Martin *The Principle of Reason* Indiana University Press 1996
Hoffmeyer, Jesper *Signs of Meaning in the Universe* Indiana 1993
Illich, Ivan *Medical Nemesis* Penguin 1990
Kay, Lily *Who Wrote the Book of Life?* Stanford University Press 2000
Kollerstrom, Nicholas *The Holocaust – Myth and Reality*
Kosok, Michael *Dialectics of Nature* Proceeding of the Telos Conference 1970
Lewontin, R.C. *Biology as Ideology, the doctrine of DNA* Harper 1993
Levin, David Michael *The Body's Recollection of Being* Routledge 1985
Maslow, Abraham *Towards a Psychology of Being* John Wiley and Sons 1968
Mindell, Arnold *Working with the Dreaming Body* Arkana 1989
McFarlane, Thomas *Integral Science* www.integralscience.org
Ronchi, Vasco *Optics, The Science of Vision* Dover 1991
Tauber, Alfred *The Immune Self: theory or metaphor?* Cambridge 1997
Wilberg, Peter *The New Medicine* (e-book) www.thenewmedicine.org.uk
Wilberg, Peter *Organismic Ontology and Organismic Healing* Energy and Character, Journal of Biosynthesis Volume 31/1
Wilberg, Peter The New Therapy (e-book) www.thenewyoga.org/TheNewTherapy.pdf
Zigmond, David *Three Types of Encounter in the Healing Arts* Journal of Holistic Medicine, April/June 1987

Also by **Peter Wilberg**

Order from amazon

The Illness is the Cure – an introduction to Life Medicine and Life Doctoring
a new existential approach to Illness

The Therapist as Listener
Martin Heidegger and the Missing Dimension of
Counselling and Psychotherapy Training

Being and Listening
Counselling, Psychoanalysis
and the Ontology of Listening

from PSYCHOSOMATICS to SOMA-SEMIOTICS -
Felt Sense and the Sensed Body in Medicine and
Psychotherapy New Yoga

Meditation and Mental Health – an introduction to
Awareness Based Cognitive Therapy

Heidegger, Phenomenology and Indian Thought

Web sites:

www.existentialmedicine.org
www.heidegger.org.uk